Chlamydia Atherosclerosis Lesion

Allan Shor

Chlamydia Atherosclerosis Lesion

Discovery, Diagnosis, and Treatment

Springer

Allan Shor, MB, ChB, M MED (Anatomical Pathology)
Johannesburg
South Africa

British Library Cataloguing in Publication Data

Shor, Allan
Chlamydia atherosclerosis lesion : discovery, diagnosis and treatment
1. Atherosclerosis 2. Chlamydia infections
I. Title
616.1'36
ISBN-13: 9781447168447

ISBN: 978-1-4471-6844-7 e-ISBN: 978-1-84628-810-4 (eBook)
DOI 10.1007/978-1-84628-810-4

Printed on acid-free paper

9 8 7 6 5 4 3 2 1

Springer Science+Business Media
springer.com

This book is dedicated to my family, who makes all the hard work worthwhile.

Preface

This book is about the atherosclerosis lesion, a lesion that blocks arteries, resulting in heart attacks, strokes, and other problems. *Chlamydia Atherosclerosis Lesion* looks at the lesion in a novel manner, through the lens of an electron microscope, where one sees a unique world, seen by very few, an ultrastructural world, showing the minutest details of how and why our arteries become blocked.

There is a need to illustrate and document these new subtle pathological findings that actually have the potential to change the concept of the disease remarkably. It is hoped that this book will stimulate interest in looking for new treatments and a cure for this dreaded disease.

It is readable by all, especially clinicians, cardiologists, neurologists, surgeons, and medical practitioners who treat this disease. Parts are readable by laymen who are interested in or suffer from the disease. There are some technical aspects concerning the pathology of the lesion, and morphological features of the *Chlamydia* germ for pathologists and microbiologists are discussed. Other topics, such as new mechanisms of lipid formation, molecular biological aspects, and new treatments, may be of value to biochemists and researchers.

Allan Shor

Contents

1 Introduction

1.1. Killer Germs That Clog Arteries

We humans are being attacked by minute killer germs that silently, stealthily, invade and clog our arteries, causing heart attacks, strokes, and other major arterial problems of pandemic proportions.

Arteries are the lifeline channels through which blood flows and is carried from the heart to all parts of the body. These can be likened to pipes or tubes. If the arteries are damaged or blocked, blood and nutrients cannot get through to supply the organs with much-needed vital substances.

The heart, itself, is supplied by three blood vessels called coronary arteries. If these become blocked and no blood passes through, then part of the heart muscle dies and a heart attack occurs.

The brain is supplied by blood via neck arteries that branch to form the cerebral arteries. Blockage of these arteries results in death of part of the brain. This is called a stroke.

The legs are supplied by iliac and femoral or leg arteries. If these arteries are blocked, then there is pain in the legs and, if the blockage is complete, death of leg muscle, or gangrene, occurs.

Blockage of other arteries, to the kidneys and bowel, also occur, causing kidney and liver problems.

Sometimes the aorta, the main artery leading from the heart, becomes damaged because of the same disease, and the artery wall becomes weakened, balloons, and bursts, usually with severe hemorrhage and death. This is called an aneurysm.

Although heart attacks, strokes, and other vascular problems are sudden, the blockage is caused by gradual production of fatty yellowish cheese-like material, called atheroma, which builds up over many years.

This blockage is widely viewed as the result of an incorrect lifestyle, overeating, overweight, lack of exercise, smoking, cholesterol, diabetes, high blood pressure, and other factors. Although these factors may be detrimental to health, the actual cause of the blockage to the arteries has recently been found to be caused by another factor, something altogether unexpected: minute killer germs that attack, destroy, and deposit in the arteries. This finding must surely rank among the most controversial of discoveries in modern times. However, there is no other way to explain the fact that when *fatty material, clogging arteries, is magnified and enlarged many thousands of times, with the aid of an electron microscope, it is seen to consist of hundreds of thousands of very small fatty germs,* and not inert cholesterol, as is widely accepted. We humans are being attacked and destroyed by minute foreign invaders and not by our own suicidal gluttonous excesses.

This book tells the story of the discovery of how these germs go about attacking, destroying, and clogging arteries, leaving a trail of destruction behind. Treatment strategies are discussed, questioning if future new medical treatments will be able to eradicate the organism, change the course of the lesion, and offer a cure of this dreaded disease.

The book is illustrated by unique and amazing photographs, micrographs, transmission electron micrographs, and scanning electron micrographs, showing an ultrastructural world of the germ and the disease as never seen before.

Let us proceed with the story by narrating the process as would be told by the germ itself. Light hearted this narration may be, but it is factual, and it introduces and sets the tone of a serious new concept of a deadly and, possibly the most common, disease in the world today.

2
The Germ's Story

2.1. A Life of Infection and Destruction

Let me introduce myself. I could best be described as a type of germ, or more precisely a bacterium, related to the *Chlamydia* family, which has been around for many generations.

It was about 20 years ago that humans found there was a clan or species of long-lost family relatives who had been overlooked all these years. They never knew of our existence until then.

After we were discovered, they decided to give us a name. In the year 1986 they called us *Chlamydia TWAR*, and then they changed the name to *Chlamydia pneumoniae*, and now to *Chlamydophila pneumoniae*.

We were first found in the eye of a child, and then they found us floating around in the air, in human respiratory passages. In the throat and lungs. They were unaware at the time we were on our way home to where we live. Inside human arteries. *We live in muscle cells in the walls of arteries, to be precise.* You see, we have to live inside these cells to survive. But please do not call us parasites. I prefer the name *obligate intracellular organism.* Sounds a bit more civilized.

We were born without certain essential metabolic mechanisms and make use of our host to supply the necessary components. We also use our host's nutrients such as fats, sugars, and proteins. These are essential for us to grow and thrive, and also to build our home. For instance, some fats are deposited in our body coverings, and other fats, such as cholesterol and phospholipids, go to help build the walls of our home.

Actually, we live in a simple home, consisting of a fatty membrane-bound vacuole that we build in our host cell. Everyone is entitled to have a home of their own, away from all unfriendly and noxious destructive agents. We thrive and multiply in our home by producing vegetative forms called reticulate bodies; these give rise to hundreds of little spore-like elementary bodies.

It is true that we finally destroy the muscle cells in which we live. But it is not our fault. How else can we multiply and grow? The vacuoles in which we live have to enlarge to accommodate all the offspring. With distension comes the inevitable, the rupture and bursting of the vacuole and, indeed, breaking up of the whole muscle cell. All the offspring are so released. We spread our offspring by dispersion. This is nature. Survival of the fittest, so they say. We may be small but we have to survive, multiply, and spread. The offspring go on to infect and live in adjacent muscle cells, and the cycle is repeated.

Of course they do not like us destroying their muscle cells in the process. *Humans have their defense mechanisms.* There are many different things that are used to try and destroy us. White blood cells come and attack us, antibodies immobilize us, and enzymes chew us up. They call this an inflammatory response. I call it weapons of mass destruction. Afterward, along come the cleaners, to clear up the mess. Scavenger cells, or macrophages as they are called. Glutinous fellows that start engulfing us and clearing the remnants of what is left over. But we are really quite sly. Even after the macrophages have eaten and engulfed us, we use all our cunning and tricks to survive.

We form nice fatty membranous vacuoles around ourselves, exactly the same as in the muscle cells. We live quite comfortably, in the vacuole, away from all harm. In the macrophages we also grow and multiply our family, same as in the muscle cells. But unfortunately, just as in the muscle cells, the scavenger macrophages also eventually rupture and demise.

This results in quite a serious mess, as one can imagine. *Large areas of necrotic cellular debris in the arterial wall, consisting of a mixture of dead cell remnants, germs, and fatty material They call this lesion "atheroma," and the disease, "atherosclerosis."* Of course, all this mess and debris cause clogging up of the artery lumen, resulting in obstruction of the blood flow. Major organs such as the heart and brain and other parts of the body simply do not get enough blood and nutrients to survive. This unhappy scenario is the cause of heart attacks, strokes, gangrene of the legs, and other vascular problems. Death of the individual is fairly common. Now, here is an interesting fact. Humans get comfort from thinking they are dying by their own hand, from lifestyle excesses. They believe there is a type of mass suicide, an epidemic of glutinous overeating and cholesterol, that is killing them.

It was not until we were spotted and recognized, caught in the act, so to say, that they even suspected we were there, let alone suspected us of causing all this upheaval. Even when we were *spotted, under an electron microscope*, lying in the messy gruel, they never recognized us. At first they said we were little blobs of fat. Now they have been getting very clever, and have started testing the fat, and they find it is not fat at all, but us germs. They have been finding our *antigens* and also our *genetic material* and even have the audacity to *grow us* in test tubes from the fatty atheroma material. Still, with all this evolving new evidence, we still do not get the full credit that we deserve. There are still questions as to our role and if we are indeed the cause of all this damage. However, if you look closely, you will see our participation in the disease.

Our participation in *muscle cell destruction*, cellular response, and gruel formation can hardly be denied.

Some form of recognition would nice. It would be appropriate to call the lesion by its rightful name, a *Chlamydia pneumoniae* infection of the arteries, rather than by the meaningless term atheroma or atherosclerosis.

If ever we are found guilty of destruction of arteries, bounty hunters will no doubt think up a few ingenious ways to bump us off. They think that if they can kill us we cannot cause damage to their arteries. What they do not know is that we have our defense systems. We just go to sleep, become dormant; become spore-like creatures, impervious to the antibiotic chemical warfare waged against us. To kill us they will need some ingenuity and find a few new antibiotics, or some more effective ones, or some combination of antibiotics. Do they really think that we are inferior or have less resistance than our friends, the tubercle bacillus or the leprosy germ, or any of the other really serious germs that cause chronic infections? Most of these chronic infectious agents require a whole arsenal of different antibiotics to kill them, and so do we.

Finally, I would like to point out there are photographs of how we live, attack, destroy, and cause the disease of atheroma. Proof that what I am telling you is true.

Here are some statistics. From surveys that test for our antibodies in blood, there is evidence that we have infected many, many, people, in different parts of the world. Also, atheroma buildup of arteries is a very common disease indeed. *This means that there are billions of us, infecting millions of people and causing disease of pandemic proportions.* It is somewhat surprising that people do not consider us really serious fellows.

3
The Deadly Disease

What we know and what we do not know about the disease

3.1. A Very Common Disease

Heart attacks, strokes, and other vascular problems are among the most common diseases in the world today. They are the result of buildup of fatty gruel deposits that clog the arteries. The name of the obstructive disease is atherosclerosis, and the actual deposits are called atheroma. It is such a common disease that it would not be amiss to state that almost every person, whether old, young, male, female, the very wealthy, or the very poor, has these lesions in their arteries, to a lesser or greater extent.

To give an indication of the frequency of this disease, it exceeds the acquired immunodeficiency syndrome (AIDS), tuberculosis, and diabetes in terms of sheer numbers of people affected. Even though heart attack incidence varies 10 fold across different nations, it is still probably the deadliest disease. Statistics published by the World Health Organization in 1996 were as follows: heart disease was the number one killer, with 7.2 million deaths; followed by cancer, 6.3 million; strokes, 4.6 million; tuberculosis, 3 million; malaria, 2.1 million; and AIDS, 1.5 million (however, this latter number has risen since then). In 1994, more than 500,000 Americans died as a result of coronary artery heart disease. It is estimated that the disease accounts for 30% to 50% of all deaths in developed nations. There are more than 32 million major atherothrombotic events worldwide each year. Atherosclerosis is an epidemic of our time [1–3].

Diagnosis of atheroma lesions, clinically, especially in persons who do not have symptoms, is difficult. A disturbing aspect is the fact that in its early stages the disease is symptom less, and people are unaware of any problem, until the deposits build up sufficiently to block the blood flowing through the arteries. Then, signs of blockage of the arteries appear. It is a well-known fact that heart attacks and strokes strike healthy people suddenly, out of the blue, without warning. Not a very cheerful thought. Early small deposits in arteries are impossible to detect, and accurate assessment of larger deposits require quite involved and special procedures and X-rays. Even with increasing advances in techniques, visualization and assessment of the lesions and the extent of the blockage in arteries is not an easy procedure that can be performed on everyone. At a meeting of vascular surgeons, someone alluded to the fact that nobody present could possibly know the locality and extent of all the atheroma deposits in their own arteries. And these are doctors who deal with the disease on a daily basis. It is just not possible to map atheroma deposits in all arteries clinically. There are very few indeed who are aware of all the deposits in their arteries, which are growing and will eventually cause obstruction of the blood supply to the heart, brain, legs, or aorta, and if they are candidates for heart attacks, strokes, vascular disease of the legs, or aortic aneurysms.

Then there is the problem of *treatment*. Even if the extent of atheroma deposits in the arteries could be determined, and with all the claims that some medication can slow progression, there is no real medical treatment that can change the course of the disease at present. The only option when symptoms of obstruction appear are surgical interventions and procedures to physically remove or bypass the blockage. But until obstruction occurs, and symptoms appear, there is little that can be done to actually prevent or reverse the progression of the disease. Preventive treatment is hampered by the fact that the medical fraternity are a bit in the dark as how to pinpoint exactly what causes the buildup of material that clogs arteries. Cholesterol, high blood pressure, smoking, and diabetes, and more than 400 other factors, have been suggested as possible causes. Stress, aging, poverty, inflammation, immunological problems, and a variety of different infections are other suggestions. In some quarters the disease is considered to be caused by a conglomerate of many factors, that is, a multifactorial disease. Preventative treatment revolves around changing one's lifestyle. The idea is to make a person healthy, decrease cholesterol in the blood, lose weight, stop smoking, bring down blood pressure, control blood sugar, exercise, and prevent stress, then hope that the buildup of the pultaceous material in the arteries will somehow cease.

However, it has been pointed out that 50% of persons who suffer heart attacks, strokes, and other vascular problems have none of the risk factors [4]. They have normal cholesterol levels in the blood, normal blood pressure, and are nondiabetics, nonsmokers, and apparently healthy persons.

One assumes that most people, especially, the very wealthy and famous, living in well-developed countries, have at their disposal and receive the very best medical attention: regular checkups, and treatment of anything amiss. If any risk factor for developing heart disease or a stroke is present, then the very best treatment is available. Cholesterol, blood pressure, and diabetes can be treated and controlled. But to no avail: blockages of arteries continue and progress over the years, silently, unabated, and continue to kill and maim [5–7]. No one is immune from this disease. Today, with all the medicines and treatments available, atherosclerosis continues as the number one disease in many parts of the world.

3.2. A Little Bit of History

It is difficult to pinpoint the very first documented case of atherosclerosis, but the disease is an old one, probably dating back to more than 5000 years, or earlier.

Egyptian mummies found in ancient pyramids of Egypt and removed from the tombs in which they were buried have been examined in some detail. Pathological findings of autopsy studies performed on some of these preserved mummies have been documented. Shattock described the presence of plaque-like lesions that were present in the arteries of an eighteenth-dynasty pharaoh, Menephthah, who was, allegedly, the Pharaoh of the Exodus. There have also been reports of several other mummies that were noted to contain similar lesions of the main arteries, including the aorta, which is the large main artery leading from the heart, the external carotid artery, which supplies the head and brain, the brachial arteries, which supply blood to the arms, and the femoral and tibial arteries, which supply the legs with blood. The features of the lesions described in the arteries are similar to the atherosclerotic lesion of today. Of course, to be sure that the lesions are the same would depend on histopathological study with assessment and interpretation of the features. Unfortunately, the tissue of the lesion after all the years is probably not suitable for electron microscopy and other types of tests that are presently available. However, from the description alone, it is reasonable to suspect that these lesions may well be similar to present-day atheroma [8–10].

Before invention of the microscope, visualization of tissue and pathological diagnosis of lesions consisted largely of macroscopic appearance, or looking at the lesion with the naked eye. In 1575 Fallopius described what he thought was degeneration of arteries into bone, and William Cowper noted that the passage of blood is impeded in some thickened arteries. Such descriptions of calcified and thickened arteries would fit in well with advanced stages of atheroma lesions that have undergone calcification, when the artery wall has become thickened with the impediment of blood flow. In 1727, a postmortem performed on a well-known doctor of the time described the finding of diseased vessels. The good doctor's arteries not only contained bone-like plaques but also the internal coat was ruptured, lacerated, and rotten. Johan Friedrich Crell emphasized pultaceous atheromatous elements of some arterial lesions. He held the view that the basal pool of material found in arteries was akin to pus and represented an endpoint of an inflammatory process. Albert von Haller was the first to apply the term atheroma to the lesion. Although it is pointed out that the term atheroma appears in the Greek literature, being a descriptive term of a cystic space containing gruel-like material, he is credited with the first use of the name atheroma.

Through the ages people have advanced certain theories as to how the lesion occurs. A blood clot that gradually forms atheromatous gruel is one theory first mooted in 1844 by Carl Von Rokatansky, who outlined his view of the disease. He described the lesion as excessive deposition of an inner vascular membrane that deposits from the blood mass. He viewed the lesion as almost like a blood clot that deposits on the inner artery and undergoes softening with formation of a fatty pultaceous mass, which later calcifies. Today, there is less enthusiasm for the theory that atheroma is an altered blood clot [8].

Virchow in 1853 viewed the lesion as a process of loosening of the connective tissue and deposition of blood constituents by a process that he described as inbibitions of the passing blood. Virchow's concept was essentially that it was not blood, but an invading stream of plasma or some moiety of the plasma, that entered the arterial wall, the so-called infiltrative theory. This phase was considered to be followed by a process of proliferation of connective tissue cells and connective tissue ground substance, followed in turn by fatty degenerative metamorphosis of connective tissue cells and formation of associated connective tissue matrix. However, the theory had its dissenters, such as Thoma in 1883, who pointed out that there were other changes that the theory did not account for, and the theory did little to explain why plasma and lipid should enter the arterial wall. However, most people seemed to supposedly like this concept, which remained a popular view of the lesion [8].

William Osler, a physician of the nineteenth century who had remarkable knowledge and medical insight, stated at the time that it is rare to find the arteries entirely free of the disease. Even in children small flecks of atheroma are by no means uncommon. After age 40 it is exceptional to examine arteries without finding this disease. He pointed to the various possible causes of this condition. One of these was simple wear and tear of life. The force exerted by blood on the artery wall, of 2.5 pounds per square inch, 100,000 times a day, must take its toll with time. The best express engine run day by day in this manner will not last one-tenth of the time of the heart's life span. He also suggested that infections and intoxications may be possible causes of the disease [11].

There are more modern theories. In 1973, Earl Benditt produced evidence that the muscle cells in atheroma were monoclonal and were derived from a very small number of precursors [12]. This hypothesis suggests that the lesion is caused in some measure by proliferation of arterial smooth muscle cells. In 1983 Benditt et al. showed viral particles to be present in some lesions of atheroma, and also in normal aorta, and postulated that the lesion could possibility be viral infective in nature [13].

In 1973, Ross and Glomset claimed proliferation of smooth muscle is the key event in the genesis of the lesion. Their study focused attention on the vascular muscle cell, as a reaction or response to some stimulus or injury of the arterial wall. Smooth muscle cell proliferation and secretion of extracellular matrix were considered responsible for developing atheroma.

In 1976 the same investigators reiterated the idea that atherosclerosis represents a "response to some type of injury." This idea went on to become a standard accepted concept of the lesion. The first step was stated to be damage to the inner lining of the artery, the endothelium. This endothelial denudation allowed fat and cells to infiltrate the artery. It was considered the initial injury was caused by shear stress, hyperlipidemia, hormone dysfunction, and other types of damage. Irrespective of injury, common responses were elicited such as smooth muscle proliferation, increased connective tissue, and lipid deposition. This classical model has not stood the test of time, and although these theories were excellent at integrating several important concepts, some of the ideas have been proven incorrect. In 1986 Ross accepted that there was no endothelial denudation of the arteries in atheroma [14]. In 1990 the lesion was viewed as a type of healing process gone awry [15] and in 1999 as an inflammatory lesion [16]. Nowadays, atheroma is proposed to be a lipid-type disease, with inflammatory and immunological molecular building blocks.

3.3. Research

No other disease comes near to being so extensively studied, in so many different ways, and by so many different disciplines, from medical practitioners to scientists to statisticians. Cardiologists study patients with atherosclerosis of the coronary arteries. Neurologists study patients with strokes caused by atheroma of arteries to the brain. Vascular surgeons deal with bypass operations for blockage of leg and other arteries, as well as arterial aneurysms. Actually, the disease is treated by many specialities; those who treat diabetes, kidney disease, and eye disease also treat and study patients with complications caused by this disease. General practitioners have their fair share of patients who suffer from atheroma. Biochemists and lipidologists appear to be the most active in study of the disease, as there is a strong belief that atherosclerosis is a lipid disease, related to cholesterol metabolism. Statisticians and epidemiologists research statistical aspects of the disease. There are many different disciplines and specialities involved in treatment and research, each with their own expertise in various different aspects. Never before has such advanced technology been available: chemical analysis, DNA testing, and unraveling of the genetic code, microscopes so powerful they can see molecules. In spite of all this, it is fair to state that mysteries and many unknowns about the disease persist.

3.4. Cholesterol

The most research evolves around cholesterol. The theory is that atherosclerosis is caused by raised serum cholesterol that infiltrates the arterial wall. James Le Fanu, in his book *The Rise and Fall of Modern Medicine* [17], points to the following. An epidemic of heart disease occurred in the 1930s and 1940s. Ancel Keys, who was an expert in nutrition, and who is well known for creating a high-calorie K ration supplement for paratroopers and American soldiers during the Second World War, focused his attention on heart attacks and atheroma after the war years. In the 1940s and 1950s, as a nutritionist he concentrated on the nutritional aspects of atheroma, especially fat and cholesterol.

Involvement of cholesterol in the disease was based on epidemiological and statistical evidence, on an observation of a general increase of heart attacks associated with a high-cholesterol diet, smoking, and high blood pressure in some parts of the world. There were criticisms, but Keys was influential, and although there was no final proof, the American Heart Association eventually endorsed the concept that lowering fat in the diet could well decrease heart attacks. However, there are studies that failed to show reduction in heart attacks by reduction of serum cholesterol, and this was and still is of some concern in acceptance of the theory [17].

This theory is a popular one and fires the imagination of the scientific community and laypersons alike. More biochemists and scientists have received Nobel prizes for cholesterol research than any other discipline in medicine. Journals of atherosclerosis are actually journals of lipid and cholesterol research. Congresses on atherosclerosis are also largely congresses on lipid and cholesterol metabolism. Text books on heart disease all contain chapters on cholesterol and the treatment thereof. The cholesterol industry is enormous, and lipid-lowering agents make up a substantial segment of the pharmaceutical industry.

Testing of cholesterol in the blood is almost mandatory for anyone visiting a doctor. A lipogram indicates the amount of cholesterol and its various different components that are present in the blood. If the cholesterol level is raised, diet or cholesterol-lowering agents are introduced. The reason given is simple enough. Cholesterol is viewed as playing a major role in the cause of heart attacks. Decreasing the cholesterol level in the blood is considered to reduce heart attacks.

In 1987 the National Cholesterol Education Program of the National Heart, Lung and Blood Institute issued guidelines and algorithms for physicians in the treatment and diagnosis of hypercholesterolemia. At approximately the same time the American Heart Association launched a physician education program aimed at placing up-to-date material in 30,000 physicians' offices, and a coronary prevention trial in hypercholesterolemic asymptomatic middle-aged men was announced [18].

The cholesterol theory relies heavily on a notion that increased serum cholesterol is a substance that infiltrates into arteries, causing clogging, and that this is the mechanism leading to heart attacks and other vascular problems [18,19].

3.5. Other Components

Although fat and cholesterol have achieved immense prominence, there are other biochemical components implicated in the lesion.

The normal artery consists of loose connective tissue with elastic and muscle cells that allow contraction of the wall to adjust to the cyclic change in pressure. Much of the connective tissue consists of carbohydrate molecules known as mucopolysaccharides or glycosaminoglycans. They are separated into nonsulfated forms such as hyaluronic acid and chondroitin, and a sulfated group of chondroitin 4-sulfate, chondroitin, and 6-sulfate and dermatan sulfate. There is an increase of these mucopolysaccharides, early in lesion formation, in fatty streaks and atherosclerotic lesions. Much research has been done on these substances, and although sophisticated chemical data and methods of studying them have evolved, there is as yet no clear understanding on the production and role of these substances in atherogenesis [20].

There are also a number of soluble proteins that can be extracted, identified, and quantitated by chemical means. These proteins include different antibodies, IgA, IgG, IgM, complement, alpha-1-antitrypsin, alpha-2-macroglobulins, fibrinogen, albumin, glycoproteins, transferrin, which is a type of iron, and ceruloplasmin. The source and reason for the presence of most of these substances are somewhat cloudy [21,22].

3.6. Molecular Biology of the Lesion

Another area of research is study of the complex molecular biological processes that take place in the lesion. For instance, there are substances that attract white cells to areas of arterial damage; these are called adhesion molecules. Then there are molecules that allow the white cells to penetrate into the artery, a mechanism that changes the infiltrated cells from monocytes to scavenger macrophages, and mechanisms for the uptake of lipid by these cells. There are actually a multitude of molecules produced by endothelial cells, smooth muscle cells, macrophages, and T-lymphocytes, as well as substances that lead to fibrosis and necrosis. Overall the molecular building blocks indicate the lesion is inflammatory and immunological in nature [23].

3.7. The Age of Statistics

There are a large number of statistical studies that examine the incidence of various different factors in patients who suffer heart attacks compared to those who do not. The attempt is to find characteristics that indicate which persons are more likely to develop a heart attack. For example, what are the chances of developing a heart attack if the blood cholesterol is raised or if blood pressure is raised? The chance of developing a heart attack in diabetics as compared to nondiabetics [24], smokers as compared to nonsmokers [25]? There are multiple other factors that have been so studied [26]: homocystine levels [27,28], growth in utero [29], low diastolic blood pressure [30], estrogen levels [31], lead [32], ceruloplasmin [33], bald men compared to those with a good head of hair [34,35], those who tall, short, fat, thin, with gray hair, black hair, age, habits, bad temper, even temper, drive cars, ride bicycles, exercise, wear black shoes, brown shoes, have increased number of earlobe creases or not. Many different types of lipids, biochemical factors, and a number of bacteria and viruses have also been so studied. In fact, much is known about the people who suffer heart attacks. Some call these factors risk factors. There are a few hundred of these risk factors that have been tied to heart attacks. One must be sensible about consideration of statistical evidence. There are many risk factors for coronary artery disease, such as snoring, gray hair, or premature baldness, that cannot comply with causality of coronary artery disease or atheroma.

In assessing the epidemiological evidence, cause must be distinguished from risk, and contributing, conditional, aggravating, and coincidental factors. Statistical correlations and parallel trends do not imply causation. In fact, Stehbens has pointed out that combining environmental, genetic, socioeconomic, and other factors may impede determination of the true causative agent in the disease [36].

3.8. Animal Studies

Then there are researchers who study atherosclerosis via animal models. These types of studies received impetus from a statement by Russell Ross in the 1980s, which stated that it may never be possible to unravel atheroma and lipid formation in humans, and that examination of the sequence of events occurring in animals that are like humans would be useful [14].

The models most relevant that have been studied are hypercholesterolemic nonhuman primates, pigtail monkeys, swine, and the WHHL (Watanabe heritable hyperlipidemic) rabbit, as well as dogs and mice. In experimental hyperlipidemic animal models, the animals are fed copious amount of fat, and the lesions that develop are characterized by lipid infiltration and large foam cells. This result has added to the concept of human atheroma being caused by lipid infiltration. There are other atherosclerotic lesions in animal models, such as those produced by trauma and various infective agents. All animal lesions are not exactly the same as those that occur in humans [37,38]. Also, it should be borne in mind that man of all the primates is uniquely affected and killed by actual arterial occlusions.

Then there are the experimental lesions that do not even need animals. Fatty material is passed through a plastic pipe until it clogs the lumen, and then solvent is passed through to open the pipe. Conclusive proof that fatty deposits clog arteries, a plumbing problem, so they say.

3.9. Modern View of the Lesion

Most studies today illustrate the atherosclerotic lesion by a series of drawings, conceptualized and based on different experimental animal models, statistical-epidemiological evidence, molecular biology, genetics, and proteomics. All the findings are intertwined and woven into a postulated disease process.

Based on a mixture of the molecular biological aspects, animal models, and statistical studies, the current concept of atherogenesis is that of an inflammatory arterial lesion formed in response to injury, by various proposed injurious agents, including lipids, homocystine, high blood pressure, and microorganisms, among others. These agents are thought to alter the properties of the endothelium and lead to a cascade of events, resulting in infiltration of various lipids and cells (blood monocytes/macrophages and T-lymphocytes), which together with proliferation of smooth muscle cells, culminates in lipid accumulation, necrosis, fibrosis, and calcification [39–41].

In the 1990s, the American Heart Association proposed a new morphological classification of atherosclerosis based on various stages of the lesion [41]. However, in spite of all we know about the lesion, the precise cause remains elusive.

References

1. Anderson RN, Kochanek KD, Murphy SL. Report of final mortality statistics, 1995. Hyattsville, Maryland: National Center for Health Statistics. Mon Vital Stat Rep 1997;45(11):suppl 2.
2. Huston SL, Lengerich EL, Conlisk E, et al. Morbidity and mortality weekly report. Centers for Disease Control. Trends in ischemic heart disease death for blacks and whites: United States, 1981–1995. JAMA 1999;281(1):28–29.
3. Henderson A. Coronary heart disease: an overview. Lancet 1996;348:S1–S2.
4. Futterman LG, Lemberg L. Fifty per cent of patients with coronary artery disease do not have any of the conventional risk factors. Am J Crit Care 1998;7(3):240–244.
5. Oliver MF. Doubts about preventing coronary heart disease. BMJ 1992;304:393–394.
6. Krumholz HM, Seeman TE, Merrill SS, et al. Lack of association between cholesterol and coronary heart disease mortality and morbidity and all cause mortality in persons older than 70 years. JAMA 1994;272:1335–1340.
7. Sacks FM, Pasternak RC, Gibson CM, et al. Effect on coronary atherosclerosis of decrease in cholesterol concentrations in normocholesterolaemic patients. Lancet 1994;344:1182–1186.
8. Woolf N. Introduction. In: Crawford T (ed) Pathology of atherosclerosis. London: Butterworth, 1982:2–4.
9. Shattock SG. A report upon the pathological condition of the aorta of King Menephtha, traditionally regarded as the Pharaoh of the Exodus. Proc R Soc Med 1909;2:122–127.
10. Sandison AT. The histological examination of mummified material. Stain Technol 1955;30:277.
11. Osler W. Diseases of the arteries. In: Fye WB (ed) William Osler's collected papers on the cardiovascular system. Birmingham: The Classics of Cardiology Library, Division of Gryphon Editions, 1985:429–433.
12. Benditt EP. Implications of the monoclonal character of human atherosclerotic plaques. Am J Pathol 1977;86(33):693–702.
13. Benditt EA, Barrett T, McDougal JK. Viruses in the etiology of atherosclerosis. Proc Natl Acad Sci U S A 1982;380:6386–6389.

14. Ross R. The pathogenesis of atherosclerosis: an update. N Engl J Med 1986; 314(8):488–500.
15. Ross R. Atherosclerosis: a defence mechanism gone awry. Am J Pathol 1993; 143(4):987–1002.
16. Ross R. Atherosclerosis: an inflammatory disease. N Engl J Med 1999;340;115–126.
17. Le Fanu J. The rise and fall of heart disease. In: Le Fanu J (ed) The rise and fall of modern medicine. London: Little Brown, 1999:322-350.
18. Gotto AM. Introduction. Symposium on hypercholesterolemia. Am J Med 1991; 91(suppl 18):1B–1S.
19. Sacks FM, Pasternak RC, Gibson CM, et al. Effect on coronary atherosclerosis of decrease in plasma cholesterol concentration in normo-cholesterolaemic patients. Lancet 1994;344:1182–1186.
20. Woodard BS, Srinivasan SR, Zimny ML, et al. Electron microscopic features of lipoprotein complexes glycosaminoglycan complexes from human atherosclerotic plaques. Lab Invest 1976;34(5):516–521.
21. Bhaki S. Complement and atherogenesis: the unknown connection. Editorial. Ann Med 1998;30:503–507.
22. Hollander W, Colombo MA, Kirkpatrick B, et al. Soluble proteins in the human atherosclerotic plaque. Atherosclerosis 1979;34:391–405.
23. Libby P. Atheroma: more than mush. Lancet 1996;348:S4–S6.
24. Ford ES, De Stafano F. Risk factors for mortality from all causes and from coronary artery disease among persons with diabetes. Findings of the national health and nutrition examination survey 1. Epidemiological follow-up study. Am J Epidemiol 1991;133:1220–1230.
25. La Rossa JC. Atherogenesis and its relationship to coronary risk factors. Clin Cornerstone 1998;1(1):3–14.
26. Harjai KI. Potential new cardiovascular risk factors: left ventricular hypertrophy, homocystine, lipoprotein(a), triglycerides, oxidative stress, and fibrinogen. Ann Intern Med 1999;131:376–386.
27. Hajjar KA. Homocystine-induced modulation of tissue plasminogen in patients with coronary artery disease. J Clin Invest 1993;10:2873–2879.
28. Winder AF. Homocystine and cardiovascular disease. Editorial. J Clin Pathol 1998;51:713–715.
29. Forsen T, Eriksson JG, Tuomilehto J, et al. Growth in utero and during childhood among women who develop coronary heart disease: longitudinal study. BMJ 1999;319:403–407.
30. Bots ML, Witteman JCM, Hoffman A, et al. Low diastolic blood pressure and atherosclerosis in elderly subjects. Arch Intern Med 1996;156:844–847.
31. Rackley CE. Estrogen and coronary artery disease in post menopausal women. Am J Med 1995;99:117–118.
32. Moller L, Kristensen TS. Blood lead as cardiovascular risk factor. Am J Epidemiol 1992;136:1091–1100.
33. Reunanen A, Knekt P, Aran R-T. Serum ceruloplasmin level and risk of myocardial infarction and stroke. Am J Epidemiol 1992;136:1082–1090.
34. Herrera CR, D'Agostino R, Gerstman BB, et al. Baldness and coronary heart disease rates in men from the Framington study. Am J Epidemiol 1995;142:828–833.
35. Wilson PWF, Kannel WS. Is baldness bad for the heart? JAMA 1993;269:1035–1036.
36. Stehbens WE. On the "cause" of tuberculosis. Pathology 1987;19:115–119.

37. Chien KR. Genes and molecular physiology in genetically engineered animals. J Clin Invest 1996;97:901–909.
38. Plump AS, Smith JD, Hyek T. Severe hypercholesterolaemia and atherosclerosis in apo-lipoprotein E deficient mice created by homologous recombination in E S cells. Cell 1992;71:343–353.
39. Hajjar DP, Nicholson AC. Atherosclerosis. Am Sci 1995;83:460–467.
40. Henderson A. Coronary heart disease: an overview. Lancet 1996;348:Si–S2.
41. Stary HC. Composition and classification of human atherosclerotic lesions. Virchows Arch Pathol Anat Histopathol 1992;421:277–290.

4
Atheroma Gruel

The mysterious membranous structures of atheroma

My involvement with study of atheroma lesions came about in the following manner. As a pathologist, my work entailed examination of large numbers of arterial specimens, which had been removed at surgical bypass operations and autopsies and then referred for further specialized study. Atheroma lesions were very common, being present in nearly every case, and very few arteries indeed were entirely free of the disease.

4.1. Study of Fatty Gruel That Clogs Arteries

The lesions varied, in severity, from small raised yellow flecks in children to large accumulations of crumbly, yellowish, cheese-like gruel material in adults, with partial or complete obstruction of the artery lumen (Figure 4.1).

The atheroma lesions when examined with a light microscope were seen to consist of nondescript fatty granular material (Figures 4.2, 4.3).

Pathologically, this fatty granular material could best be described as a focus of fatty necrotic gruel in the artery.

There are a variety of different agents that can potentially cause death of tissue or necrosis. Chemicals, toxins, germs, radiation, and decreased blood supply are some possibilities. A few microscopic studies were undertaken to try and find the elusive agent, but to no avail. No sign of poisons, toxins, infective agents, or blood clots in the small nutritive vessels could be found to account for the lesion.

Not only the cause but also the nature of the necrotic material was *shrouded in mystery*. Was it necrosis of the artery wall or necrosis of an infiltrate of fat, inflammatory cells, or other substances? Special stains were used to examine necrotic atheroma material, and use was also made of an instrument that was capable of analyzing the chemical constituents of tissue. Analysis indicated that much fat, as well as mucopolysaccharides, collagen, calcium, iron, and other chemical constituents, were present. Unfortunately this information did not bring understanding of the origin of the necrotic material nearer.

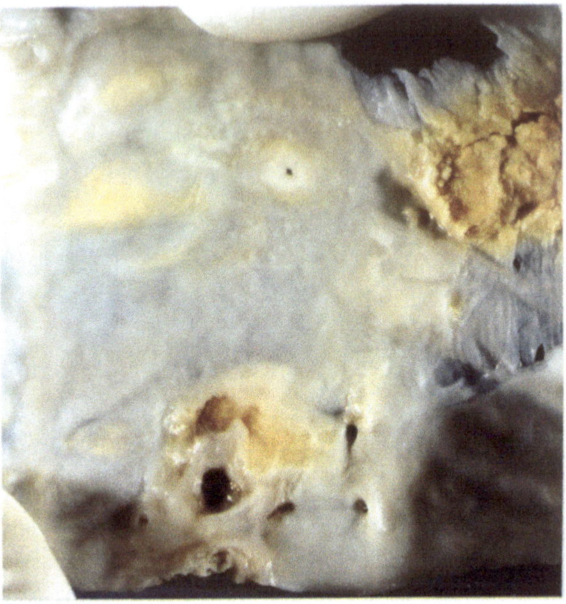

Figure 4.1. Atheroma gruel. Opened artery, spread flat to illustrate two foci of yellowish crumbly atheroma gruel in the artery wall. This is the killer substance that clogs arteries.

An ordinary light microscope cannot show structures smaller than the wavelength of light. Magnification is limited to 1250 times maximum. To determine the contents of the necrotic gruel in more detail, much greater magnification is required. For this, it is necessary to use a special type of microscope, an *electron microscope*, capable of visualizing ultrastructure and even molecular components.

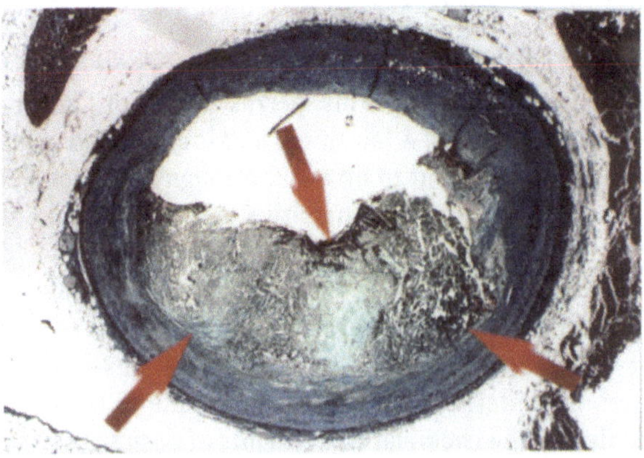

Figure 4.2. Atheroma gruel blocking artery. Micrograph shows transverse section of artery with atheroma gruel partially obstructing artery lumen (area enclosed with *arrows*).

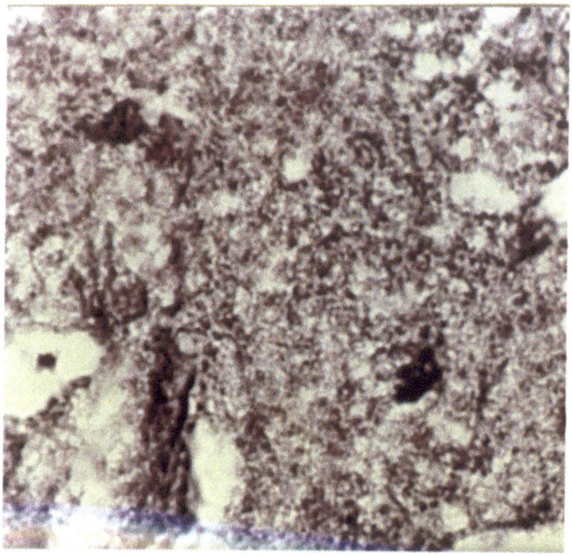

FIGURE 4.3. Atheroma gruel seen under microscope. Micrograph shows atheroma gruel. Cut a small slice of necrotic gruel material, fix it in formalin, process in alcohols, and then embed in a wax block. Cut a section 5 micrometers (μm) thick. Put the section on a glass slide and stain, add a coverslip, and examine the gruel with a light microscope at 1000× magnification. This is what is seen: nondescript granular fatty material.

4.2. Electron Microscope

This is not an ordinary piece of equipment. Even delivery and transportation of a new electron microscope, from the delivery truck in the parking bay to the second floor of the building where I worked and where the instrument was to be housed, was a major feat in itself. The microscope weighed a few tons and, after delivery, the floor housing the instrument had to be reinforced to hold such a heavy weight. I was thankful for this consideration, as my office was on the floor below. It took a few months for installation of the instrument, but toward the end of the year of 1989, a new powerful electron microscope was fully functional and ready for use (Fig. 4.4).

Here are some details of this type of microscope. Instead of light, the instrument uses electromagnets to focus a beam of electrons in a vacuum. Because the wavelength of electrons is much smaller than that of light, an electron microscope is capable of magnifying tissue up to a million times normal size, and its resolving power is 250,000 finer than the human eye. At 100,000-fold magnification, a tissue 1 millimeter (mm) in size is enlarged to the size of a football field, and one can see cellular ultrastructural detail and visualize small germs and viruses. If the tissue is magnified a million times, molecular detail starts becoming visible. The electron microscope is limited in that cells and

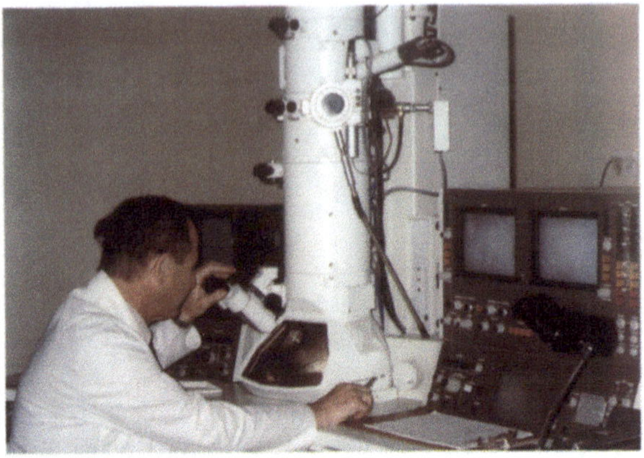

FIGURE 4.4. Electron microscope. An electron microscope is a large complicated piece of equipment that uses electrons instead of light to magnify tissue many thousands of times.

tissue cannot survive in a vacuum and so the instrument cannot show movements of living cells.

Preparation of tissue for electron microscopy requires specialized processing. Small pieces of atheroma tissue are removed from the arteries and placed in small bottles containing special fixative. The tissue is then processed and embedded in a special plastic material. Thin slivers of tissue are cut from the blocks, placed on special small copper grids, and stained. The grids are then inserted into a special container in the electron microscope for viewing. The image is projected onto a screen and viewed through a special glass-covered window.

To illustrate the intensity and time that is required to examine tissue, one needs to consider that the screen on which the electron microscopic image is viewed measures about 20 centimeters (cm) in diameter. To examine tissue enlarged to the size of a football field, 20 cm^2 at a time, gives some indication of the time-consuming effort that is required. Examination of tissue in such detail takes many hours, and a single atheroma lesion could well take a few days of examination, in some cases.

4.3. Electron Microscopic Features of Atheroma Gruel

The following is what was seen when atheroma gruel was examined with an electron microscope.

Fatty atheroma gruel consists of a conglomerate of hundreds of thousands of little membranous structures. Some are round, some irregular, and some are pear shaped. The size varies between 100 and 600 nanometers (nm; a nanometer is a millionth of a millimeter). Some contain dense material, and some show budding, dividing, and sporulating forms.

The electron microscopic features of the structures in atheroma gruel appear different to conventional fat. They consist of tightly packed membranous structures.

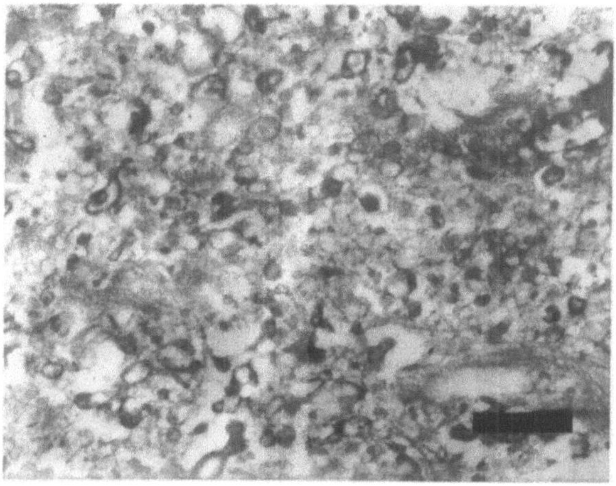

Figure 4.5. Transmission electron micrograph of atheroma gruel. A conglomerate of dense membranous structures that are tightly packed together. What are these structures that make up the atheroma gruel?

I studied the various structures in detail. Photographs were taken; negatives were developed, enlarged, and printed. The printed electron micrographs were further examined, and each of the fatty membranous structures was scrutinized in even greater detail with the aid of a magnifying glass (Figures 4.5–4.18).

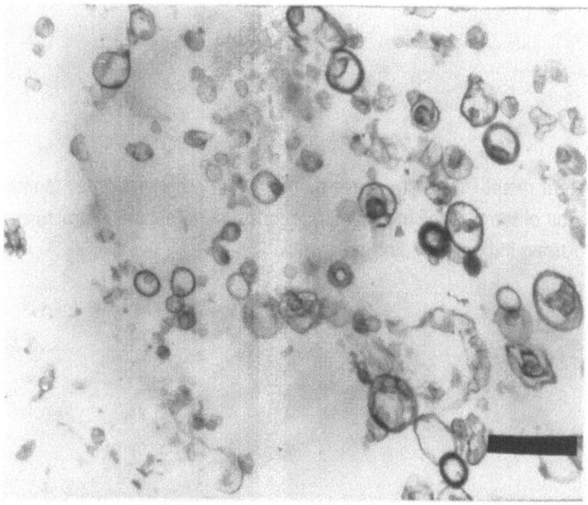

Figure 4.6. Transmission electron micrograph of atheroma gruel. Less dense area, showing contents of small membranous structures of various sizes and shapes. Some are budding and some are dividing. *Bar* 400 nm.

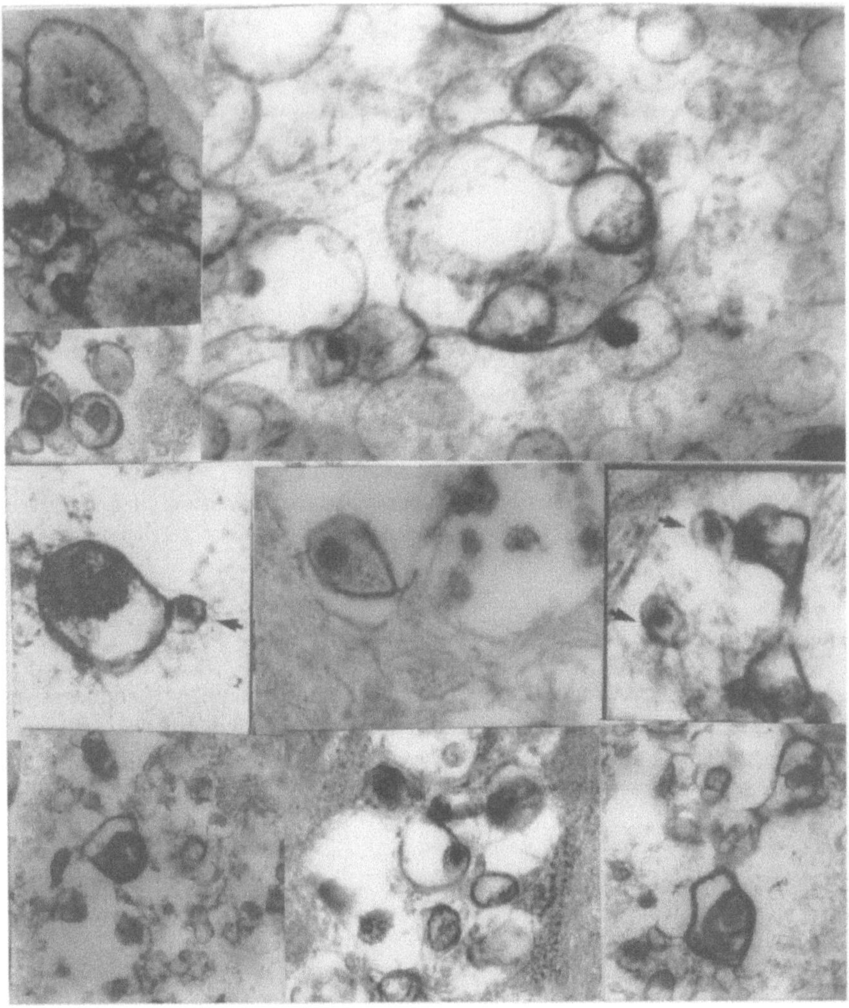

Figure 4.7. Different membranous structures that make up atheroma gruel. Montage electron micrograph of a collection of some of the many different forms of membranous structures that were found in atheroma gruel. Arrows indicate budding structures.

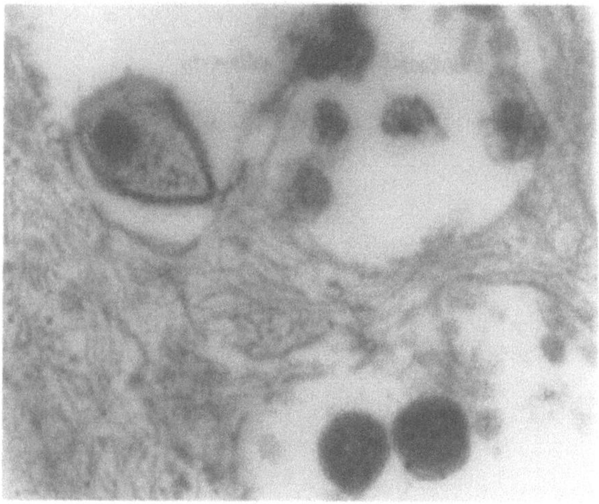

Figure 4.8. Pear-shaped and dense structures. Pear-shaped structure contains electron-dense material and is enclosed with bilamellar membrane. Also, smaller electron-dense structures are present.

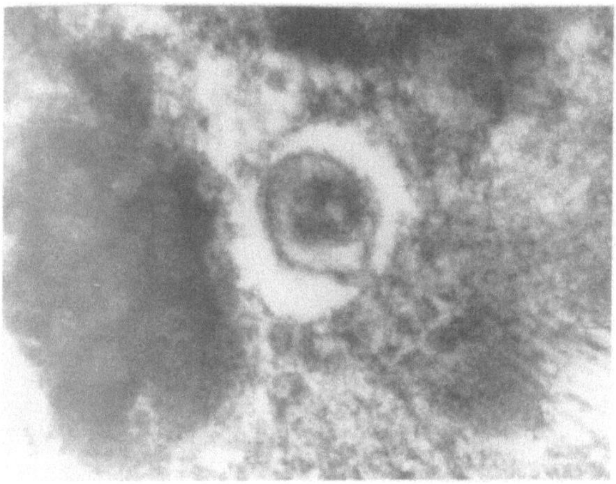

Figure 4.9. Pear-shaped structure containing electron-dense material in vacuole.

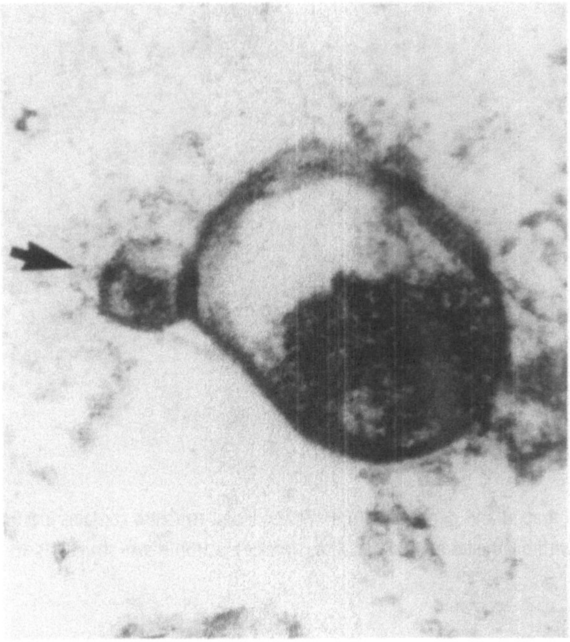

Figure 4.10. Budding structure. Structure containing electron-dense material and showing membranous budding (*arrow*).

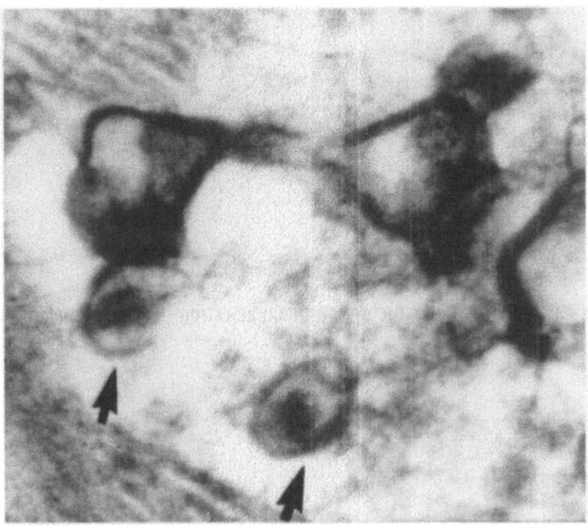

Figure 4.11. Dividing structures. Two pear-shaped dividing structures contain electron-dense material and membranous budding (*arrows*).

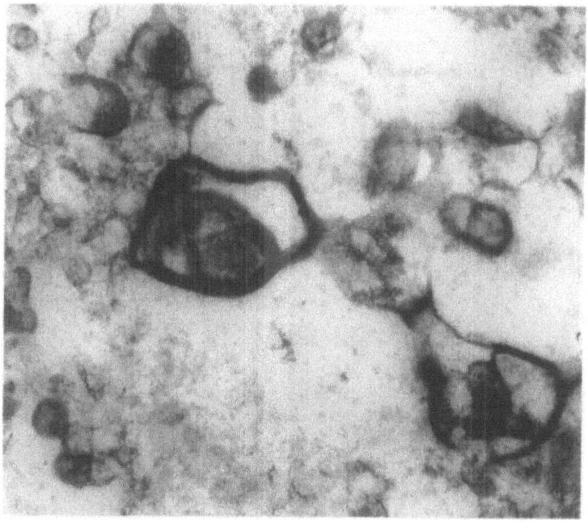

Figure 4.12. Dividing structures. Structure dividing into three.

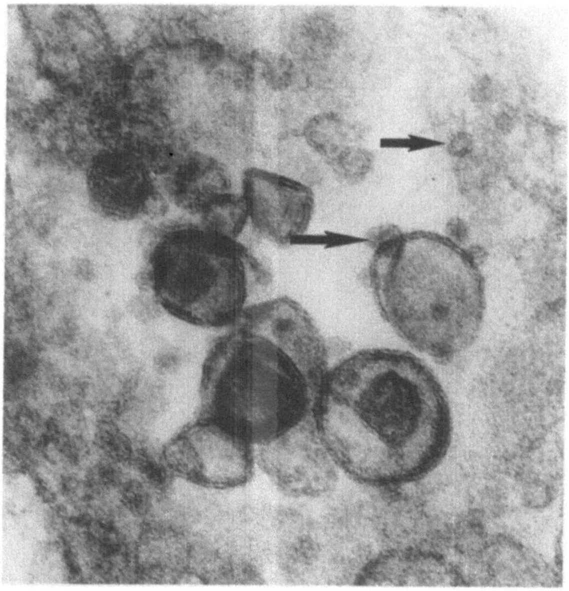

Figure 4.13. Membrane blebs. A collection of round and pear-shaped membranous structures with small membrane blebs (*arrows*).

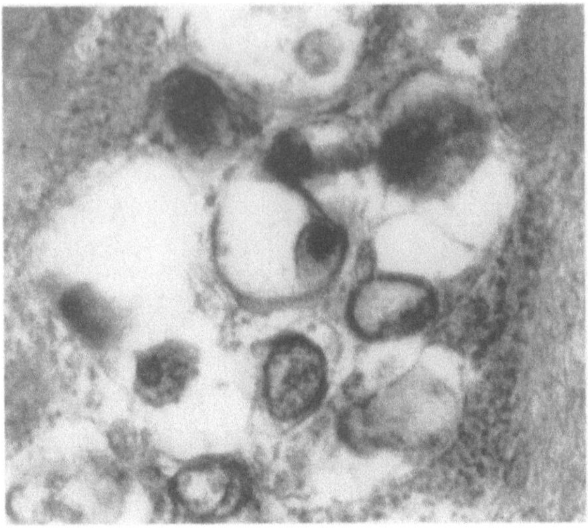

Figure 4.14. Sporulating forms. Round membranous structures with a pear-shaped structure in a vacuole.

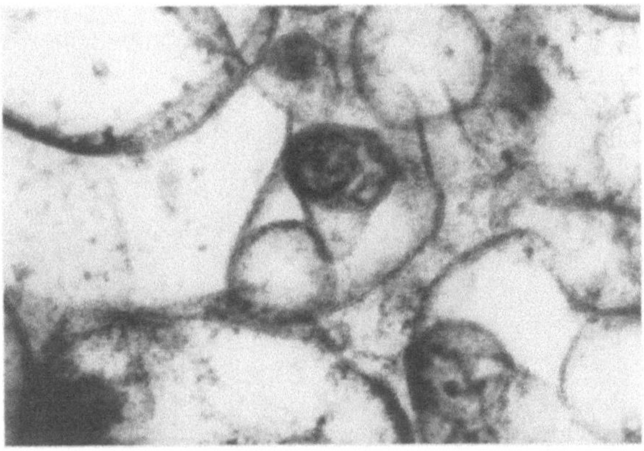

Figure 4.15. Sporulating forms. Sporulating structures, one of which is pear shaped.

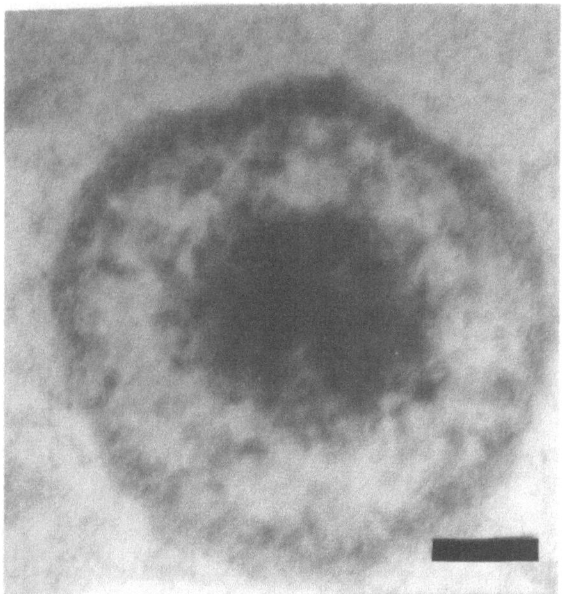

Figure 4.16. Round structures. Round structure with central dense material. *Bar* 100 nm.

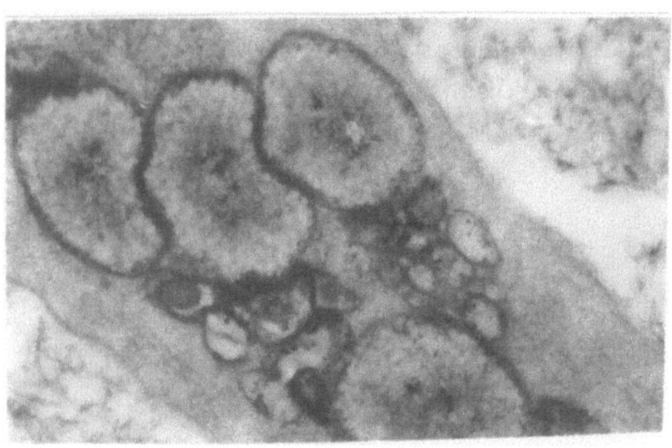

Figure 4.17. Round crenated structures. Round crenated membrane-bound structures with central dense material, and fine radiating reticulate material. Smaller grape-like budding structures are present.

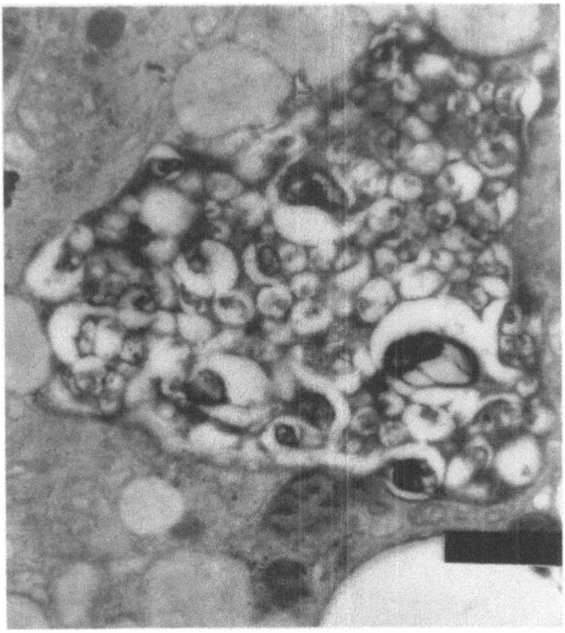

Figure 4.18. Multiple germs in vacuole. Transmission electron micrograph of intracellular vacuole containing multiple small membranous structures of different sizes and shapes.

What are these membranous structures that make up atheroma gruel, where do they come from, and how are they formed?

5
Discovery

See what everyone sees but think what no one thinks

Looking through the literature, I came across some articles on electron microscopic findings of human atherosclerotic lesions. The various structures described bore some similarity to what I had noted in atheroma.

The articles illustrated and described atheroma gruel as a lipid-rich core consisting of a collection of membranous lipid structures in the form of small lipid droplets, vesicles, dense bodies, and unknown bodies. These structures were thought to be derived from serum lipids that had undergone physicochemical change [1–12].

There were, however, some problems with accepting an explanation of derivation of structures from serum lipids. For instance, by electron microscopy, no fat is present in the superficial part of the artery, as one would expect if the fat infiltrated from serum. Accumulation of lipid structures occurs in the deeper part of the artery. Then, there is the fact that the fat structures of atheroma contain types of fat that are different from those in serum. Also, the pathological features of gruel are more like necrotic material rather than simple fat.

I examined the electron micrographic features of the structures that I had found in atheroma gruel, over and over again, with a magnifying glass. Looking at more and more electron microscopic features of the membranous structures, a new thought entered my mind. A new possibility opened up. *Electron-dense structures* enclosed with double membranes, which multiply, divide, bud, and sporulate, do not look like conventional fat, but *have features more suggestive of some type of living, growing microorganism.*

5.1. Does Atheroma Gruel Consist of Fat or Germs?

Could the fatty membranous structures in atheroma really be some type of minute, living fatty microbe? *A germ?* An organism so small and devious that it has escaped discovery and identification, being mistaken for blobs of fat, over all the years?

Fat is fat and germs are germs. How could the two be confused with each other? But on reading about germs and fats in microbiological and biochemistry textbooks, it was noted that many germs contain various fats and cholesterols, use fats, and produce fats. Indeed, based on appearance and fat content, the membranous structures in atheroma could well be fatty germs.

5.2. Which Germ?

Which germ could it possibly be? One method to identify a germ is by its physical appearance. Every germ has its own unique characteristic features, the same as creatures in the macro-world. For example, there are general features that separate humans from animals, and also specific features identifying individuals. The same principles apply to the germ kingdom. Features of germs are invaluable for identification.

I made a drawing of all the sizes, shapes, contents, membranes, budding, dividing, sporulating, and whatever I noticed about the fatty structures in atheroma lesions. Then with a collection of the electron micrographs, drawings, and measurements, I strolled to the medical library, selected a few nice big detailed microbiology books from the shelf [13–16], and started paging through the books and literature looking at the pictures and descriptions of microorganisms, viruses, bacteria, fungi, and protozoa. I particularly studied the electron microscopic morphological features of the various germs.

Was there an organism with similar features that could compare to the photographs and drawings of the structures I had seen in atheroma lesions?

The structures were too small to be fungi and protozoa. At first I thought the structures may possibly be large viruses. Viruses vary in size. The smallest are roughly 30 nm and the largest up to 500 nm in size. Most are in the range of 100 to 200 nm. The structures in atheroma were between 100 and 600 nm with some larger structures a few micrometers in size.

There had been articles in the early 1980s suggesting that herpes-type viruses may be present in atheroma and also in normal arteries. However, morphological features of the different types of virus particles in books did not show similar features to structures I had seen in atheroma gruel. Then, on to study the morphological features of bacteria. Most of the electron micrographs of bacterial microorganisms showed much larger forms, some containing a variety of organelles, totally different to that which I had noted in atheroma. However, there were some groups of bacteria, the *Mycoplasmataceae*, *Rickettsiaceae*, *Chlamydiaceae*, and *Bartonellaceae* group, that had some possible similarities. More study of these particular bacteria showed that *Rickettsiaceae* were elongated and consisted of forms differing from those present in atheroma structures. *Mycoplasmataceae* were in a variety of forms, some with similar features, but these organisms did not have an intracellular life cycle and also no larger forms. I spent a lot of time looking at *Bartonellaceae*. These are red blood cell pathogens. I drew some articles on the germ [17]. In the end I concluded that even though the germ had similar intracytoplasmic features, there was no comparable life cycle.

Chlamydia, *on the other hand, were of similar size, with similar features, and had a similar intracellular life cycle.* There were small elementary bodies and larger vegetative reticular forms. Growth is in vacuoles in the host cell cytoplasm, and spread is by rupture of host cells with dispersion, similar to that which was noted to occur to structures of atheroma. *Chlamydia* organisms contain 30% to 50% of lipid consisting of various fatty acids, triglycerides, phospholipids, and 7.5% cholesterol. This description fits in well with the lipid content of atheroma.

5.3. A *Chlamydia* Germ

Microbiology books contained a list of various reference articles on electron microscopic features of different *Chlamydia* organisms and species [18–29].

Looking through these, I came across an article written by Armstrong et al. in 1963 on the electron microscopic features of a cultured *Chlamydia* trachoma agent isolated from the eye. *The article described and contained micrographs of various forms of the organism. One of the plates, number 6, showed pictures of elementary forms of* Chlamydia *germs that were uncanny in their similarity to the structures which had been seen in atheroma* [18]. My heart missed a beat. The structures were pear shaped and dividing, exactly the same as in atheroma. Also, larger reticulate forms were identical to some of the larger lipid structures found in atheroma (Figures 5.1–5.4).

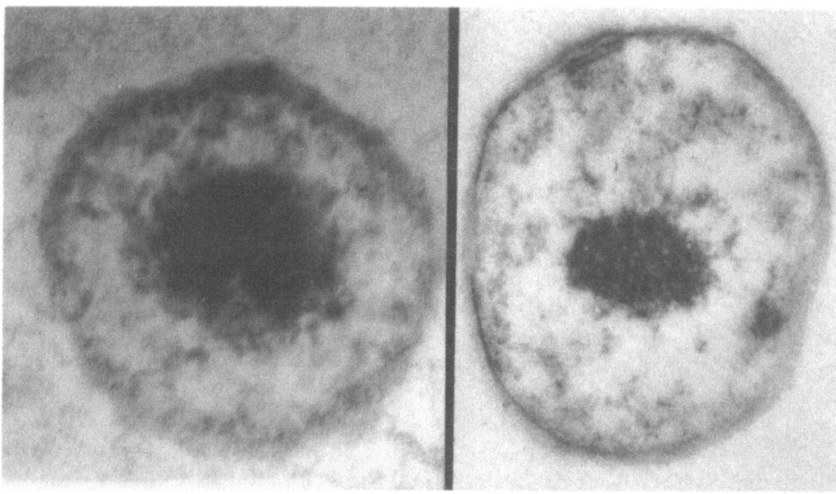

Figure 5.1. Transmission electron micrographs of atheroma structure (*left*) compared to cultured *Chlamydia* organism (*right*). Both are round and contain central dense material and are enclosed by an outer membrane. (From Armstrong JA, Valentine RC, Fildes C [18], with permission of the *Journal of General Microbiology*.)

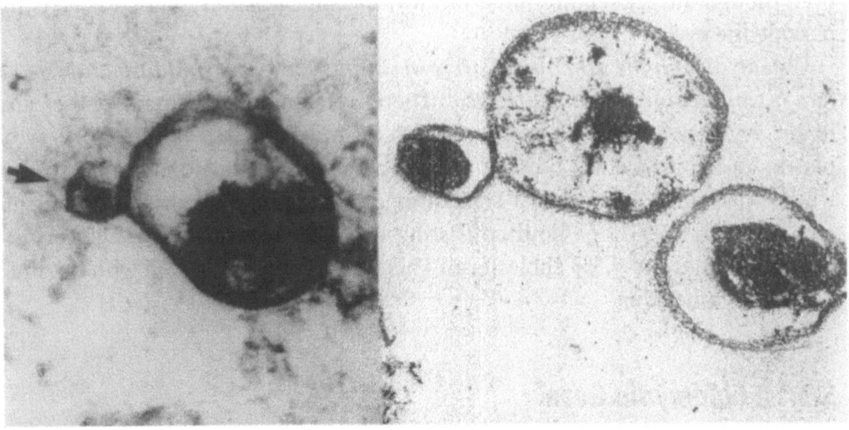

Figure 5.2. Transmission electron micrographs of atheroma structure (*left*) compared to cultured *Chlamydia* organism (*right*). The structures are similar. Both contain dense material, are membrane bound, and show similar membranous budding. (From Armstrong JA, Valentine RC, Fildes C [18], with permission of the *Journal of General Microbiology*.)

I went on to look at all the articles on the electron microscopic features of *Chlamydia* organisms that I could find. An article by Manor and Sarov showed pictures of *degenerate* Chlamydia *germs in macrophages that were similar to degenerate membranous structures in atheroma* [25]. Articles in other journals described *miniature forms* [29]. In fact, there were many articles on the

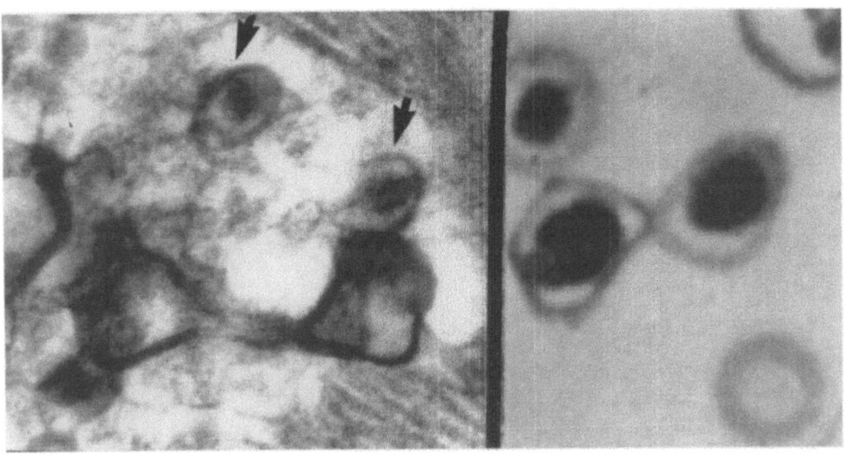

Figure 5.3. Transmission electron micrographs of atheroma structure (*left*) and cultured *Chlamydia* organism (*right*). Both show similar division and pear-shaped structures with electron-dense material and budding structures. Arrows indicated budding structures. (From Armstrong JA, Valentine RC, Fildes C [18], with permission of the *Journal of General Microbiology*.)

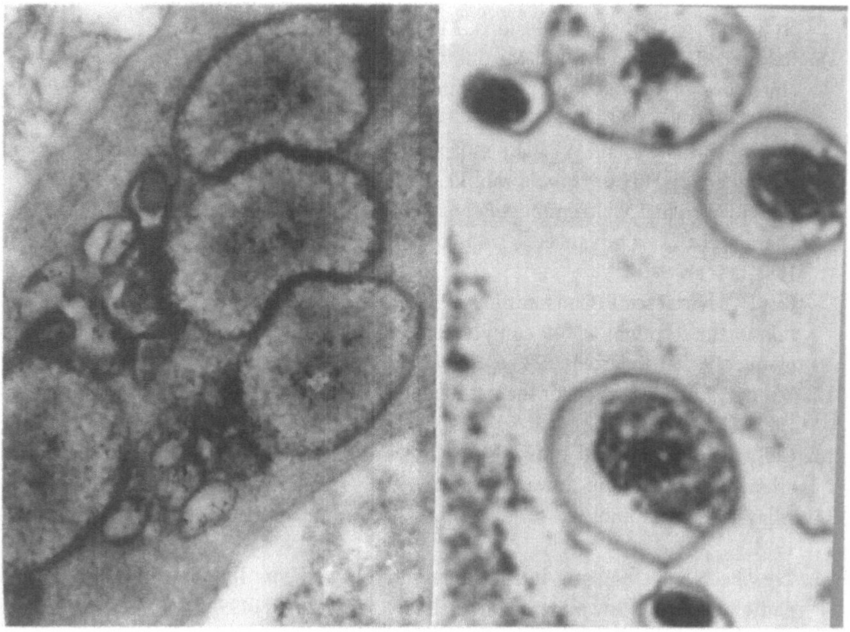

Figure 5.4. Transmission electron micrographs showing atheroma structures(*left*) compared to cultured *Chlamydia* organism (*right*) Structures are roundish in shape with electron-dense material, and show outer membrane budding. (From Armstrong JA, Valentine RC, Fildes C [18], with permission of the *Journal of General Microbiology*.)

morphological features of Chlamydia *germs that bore some similarity to the structures I had seen in atheroma* [18–29].

References

1. Bocan TMA, Schifani TA, Guyton JR. Ultrastructure of the human aortic fibrolipid lesion. Formation of the atherosclerotic lipid-rich core. Am J Pathol 1986;123: 413–424.
2. Chao F-F, Amende LM, Blanchete-Mackie EJ, et al. Unesterified cholesterol-rich particles in atherosclerotic lesions of human and rabbit aortas. Am J Pathol 1988; 131(1):73–83.
3. Geer JC, McGill HC Jr, Strong JP. The fine structure of human atherosclerotic lesions. Am J Pathol 1961;3(38):263–287.
4. Geer JC. Fine structure of aortic intimal thickening and fatty streaks. Lab Invest 1965;4:1764–1783.
5. Guyton JR, Klemp KF. The lipid-rich core of human atherosclerotic fibrous plaques. Prevalence of small lipid droplets and vesicles by electron microscopy. Am J Pathol 1989;134(3):705–717.
6. Guyton JR, Klemp KF. Transitional features in human atherosclerosis. Am J Pathol 1993;143(5):1444–1457.

7. Hoff HH. Human intracranial atherosclerosis. A histochemical and ultrastructural study of gross fatty streak lesions. Am J Pathol 1972;69:421–438.
8. Rekhter MD, Andreeva ER, Mironov AA, Orekhov AN. Three-dimensional cytoarchitecture of normal and atherosclerotic intima of human aorta. Am J Pathol 1991;138(3):569–580.
9. Rogers KM, Stehbens WE. The morphology of matrix vesicles produced in experimental arterial aneurysms in rabbits. Pathology 1986;18:64–71.
10. Ross R, Wright TN, Strandness E, et al. Human atherosclerosis cell constitution and characteristics of advanced lesions of the superficial femoral artery. Am J Pathol 1984;114(1):79–92.
11. Rus HG. Nicelescu F, Constantinescu E, et al. Immunoelectron-microscopic localisation of the terminal C5b-9 complement complex in human atherosclerotic fibrous plaques. Atherosclerosis 1986;61:35–42.
12. Watts HF. Basic aspects of the pathogenesis of human atherosclerosis. Hum Pathol 1971;2(1):31–55.
13. Collier LH. Topley and Wilson's principles of bacteriology, virology and immunity, 8th ed, vol 2. London: Edward Arnold, 1990.
14. Atlas RM. Microbiology fundamentals and applications. New York: Macmillan, 1984.
15. Cheville NF. Pathogenic intracellular microorganisms. In: Cheville NF (ed) Cell pathology. Ames: Iowa State University Press, 1976:474–499.
16. Schachter J. *Chlamydia.* In: Goebel W (ed) Current topics in microbiology and immunology, vol 138. Intracellular bacteria. Heidelberg: Springer–Verlag, pp 109–133.
17. Ristic M, Kreier JP. Hemotropic bacteria. N Engl J Med 1979;301(17):937–939.
18. Amstrong JA, Valentine RC, Fildes C. Structure and function of the trachoma agent in cell cultures as shown by electron microscopy J. Gen Microbiol 1963;30:359–373.
19. Doughri AM, Storz J, Altera KP. Mode of entry and release of chlamydiae in infections of intestinal epithelial cells. J Infect Dis 1972;126:652–657.
20. Friss RR. Interaction of L cells and *Chlamydia psittaci.* Entry of the parasite and host responses to its development. J Bacteriol 1972;110:706–721.
21. Hackstead T, Fischer ER, Scidmore MA, et al. Origins and function of the chlamydial inclusion. Trends Microbiol 1997;15(7):288–289.
22. Hodinka R, Wyrick PB. Ultrastructural study of mode of entry of *Chlamydia psittaci* into L929 cells. Infect Immun 1986;54(3):855–863.
23. Hodinka RL, Davis CH, Choong J, Wyrick PB. Ultrastructural study of endocytosis of *Chlamydia trachomatis* by McCoy cells. Infect Immun 1988;56(6):1456–1463.
24. Wyrick PB, Choong J, Davis CH, et al. Entry of genital *Chlamydia trachomatis* into polarized human epithelial cells. Infect Immun 1989;57(8):2378–2389.
25. Manor E, Sarov I. Fate of *Chlamydia trachomatis* in human monocytes and monocyte derived macrophages. Infect Immun 1986;54(1):90–95.
26. Moulder JW. The chlamydial inclusion membrane as an engine of survival. (Letter.) Trends Microbiol 1997;5(8):305–306.
27. Peterson EM, de la Maza LM. *Chlamydia* parasitism. Ultrastructural characterization of the interaction between the chlamydial cell envelope and the host cell. J Bacteriol 1998;170(3):1389–1392.
28. Raulston JE. Micro review. Chlamydial envelope components and pathogen–host cell interaction. Mol Microbiol 1995;15.(4):607–616.
29. Tanami Y, Yamada Y. Miniature cell formation in *Chlamydia psittaci.* J Bacteriol 1973;114:408–412.

6 Which *Chlamydia* Species?

A search for the culprit

6.1. Some Unique Features of the *Chlamydia* Germ in Atheroma

Germs in atheroma show common features to *Chlamydia* organisms, but there are some differences.

Structures with central dense material, reticular radiations, and dividing and budding forms are similar to other *Chlamydia*, but *sporulation is a unique feature of the atheroma germ.* Also, scarcity of organisms, atypical forms, and ghost forms (where the germ has no contents) typify the elementary organism in atheroma.

In cell culture, the life cycle has been restricted to intracellular aspects, whereas in *atheroma lesions, the extracellular life cycle*, after cell rupture and dispersion, is a prominent feature. Outside the cell, further growth, division, and budding of the germs take place. This cycle has not been previously described.

A peculiar feature of the atheroma organism concerns the vacuole in which the organisms grow and multiply. *The vacuole persists and also enlarges and grows extracellularly in atheroma gruel* following rupture of the host cell. This feature of *Chlamydia* has not been described.

There has always been controversy as to whether the *Chlamydia* parasitephorous vacuole, in which the organisms grow, is part of the organism or part of the host cell. The reason for this dilemma is because the vacuole is formed from the host's cellular membrane and therefore is part of the host. However, strangely enough, it undergoes changes and starts producing *Chlamydia* organisms.

Finding an independent extracellular existence of the vacuolar membrane suggests the possibility that the vacuole may become part of the organism rather than remain as part of the host cell (Table 6.1).

TABLE 6.1. Features of *Chlamydia* in atheroma compared to cultured *Chlamydia*

	Atheroma	Culture
INTRACELLULAR GROWTH OF *CHLAMYDIA*	Grow in vacuoles in muscle cells and macrophages	Grow in cytoplasmic vacuoles in various cell cultures, including He La cells, aortic endothelium, muscle, and macrophages
RETICULATE FORMS	1. Fibrillar forms, with central dense core and limiting membrane 2. Sporulating and budding forms	1. Large membrane-bound forms, sometimes fibrillar forms with dense core 2. Divide by binary fission 3. Intermediate forms
ELEMENTARY FORMS	1. Pleomorphic with various different shapes 2. Round and pear-shaped forms with large periplasmic space, occasionally with dense bodies and membrane blebs 3. Dense forms 4. Atypical forms and ghost forms common	1. Pleomorphic and various shapes 2. Round and pear-shaped forms, with large periplasmic space, miniature bodies, and membrane blebs (TWAR) 3. Dense forms (TWAR)
EXTRACELLULAR CYCLE	1. **ELEMENTARY FORMS** Typical and atypical forms Occasional dividing, budding, and miniature forms 2. **RETICULATE BODIES** Unusual; seen only after cell rupture 3. **VACUOLAR MEMBRANES** Appear to enlarge and grow, after cell rupture	Not described in cell culture

6.2. Not Conventional *Chlamydia* Species

What special type of *Chlamydia* could the atheroma germ be? Perhaps reading about *Chlamydia* germs could offer some insight as to what we are considering.

Chlamydia germs have been around for a long time. They were known by various names, such as Eaton's agent, *Bedsonia*, *Chlamydozoaceae*, and *Miyagawanella*. In 1907, Halberstaedter and Von Prowaseck were the first to describe transmission of the germ, from humans to orangutans, via eye scrapings. In Giemsa-stained conjunctival epithelial cells, they found intracytoplasmic inclusions containing numerous minute particles, now known as elementary bodies, and concluded correctly that these represented the causal agent of the disease [1].

Soon afterward, similar infections were diagnosed in babies and also in cases of urethritis in adult males. In 1929–1930, widespread outbreaks of psittacosis or pneumonia transmitted from birds occurred, and these were found to be caused by similar germs. About this time, a similar agent causing lymphogranuloma venereum, a venereal disease, was first propagated in monkey brain and then in chick embryos. They all formed a unique group that were considered as "atypical viruses." They live in cells, require host nutrients for survival, and could not be cultured in an artificial medium. These are characteristics of viruses.

A major understanding of *Chlamydia* was achieved by Moulder (1964), who marshalled compelling evidence for regarding these agents as bacteria and not atypical viruses. As the organisms are able to survive outside the cells, they were classified as bacteria. Bacteria are germs that have cell walls and an independent survival. *Chlamydia* are therefore now classified as obligate intracellular bacteria [1].

Two types of *Chlamydia* were described at the time: one is a *Chlamydia* sp. of which there are different strains causing various different infections, such as eye infections and sexually transmitted disease; the other species is a *Chlamydia* responsible for lung infection or pneumonia that is transmitted by various birds and other pets and has also occurred in turkey and duck processing plants because of droplets carried in from dust in feathers or from dry fecal material [1].

The atheroma germ did not seem to be related to either of these species. Arterial disease was not more common in people who had sexually transmitted disease or eye infections or those in contact with birds. Also, the morphological features of the organisms differed in some respects.

6.3. A New *Chlamydia* Species

In the late 1980s, journals and microbiology textbooks were starting to introduce information on a new *Chlamydia* species in humans [1–5]. In 1980, Darouger et al. (as cited in Collier) had reported that 20% of blood donors in London possessed antibody to an *atypical* Chlamydia *(IOL-207)* that had been first isolated in Iran, from a child.

There were also reports in the mid-1980s concerning epidemics of mild pneumonia that had occurred in two Northern Finish communities and four military garrisons. Serological studies of these patients suggested that an unusual strain of *Chlamydia psittaci* caused the epidemic. However, as it was wintertime and no birds were around, the infection could not have been by avian transmission. Furthermore, *Chlamydia* antibody tests were negative for *Chlamydia trachomatis* and the conventional *psittaci* strain, but with further testing it was found to be positive for a special *Chlamydia psittaci* strain, TW-183, which had first been isolated in 1965 in Taiwan from the eye of a primary-school child with trachoma. The strain was similar to IOL-207, which had also been isolated from the eye of a trachoma patient in Iran. Despite the conjunctival source of isolates of both strains, serological testing suggested the organisms were not related to eye disease. In 1983, a similar isolate was obtained from a student at the University of Washington with an upper respiratory tract throat infection. The isolate was called AR-39, and so a new strain of *Chlamydia* was established in 1987 with the name *TWAR*, a combination of the names for strains TW-183 and AR-39. The strains were first classified as a *Chlamydia psittaci* strain by Kuo et al. on the basis of inclusion morphology and lack of glycogen.

Later, Cox et al. found only 10% homology between TWAR agents and *Chlamydia trachomatis* and *Chlamydia psittaci*. Also, the TWAR strain contained no plasmid. Furthermore, the elementary forms differed in morphology in being pear shaped with a large periplasmic space, within which are round electron-dense bodies 50 nm in diameter attached to the cytoplasm by string-like structures. Grayston suggested that *Chlamydia* TWAR be classified as a new species, which was called *Chlamydia pneumoniae* in 1989.

The new *Chlamydia* germs had been cultured, and there were articles with electron micrographs on the morphological features of the new germs grown in culture.

The electron micrographs of the germ in culture compared favorably with the structures that had been noted in atheroma. *The elementary pear-shaped membranous structures with membrane blebs of* Chlamydia *TWAR were similar to some of the lipid structures of atheroma. Also, the round dense structures as seen in cultured* Chlamydia *IOL207 were similar to the small dense bodies seen in atheroma* (Figures 6.1–6.4).

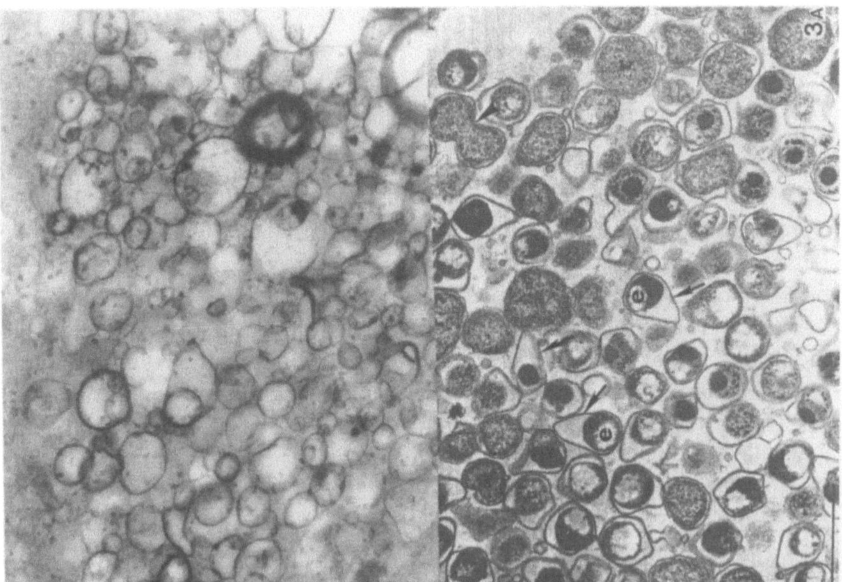

Figure 6.1. Atheroma structures compared to *Chlamydia* TWAR Round and pear-shaped *Chlamydia* organisms of atheroma (*left*) compared to round and pear-shaped structures of cultured *Chlamydia* TWAR organisms (*right*). Similar structures, but some atheroma structures contain no contents and consist of outer membranes only. (Electron micrograph for comparison from Chi et al. [6], with permission from the *Journal of Bacteriology*.)

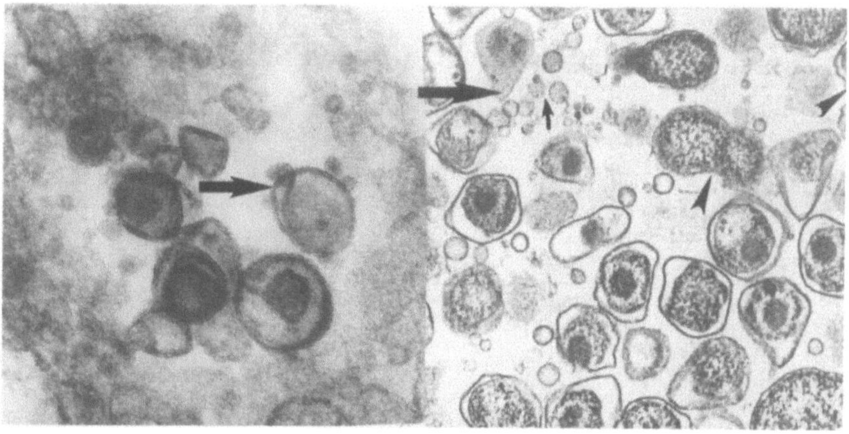

Figure 6.2. Atheroma structures compared to *Chlamydia* TWAR Atheroma structures (*left*) with membrane blebs (*arrows*) compared to cultured *Chlamydia* TWAR (*right*) with membrane blebs (*arrowhead*). (Electron micrograph for comparison from Chi et al. [6], with permission from the *Journal of Bacteriology*.)

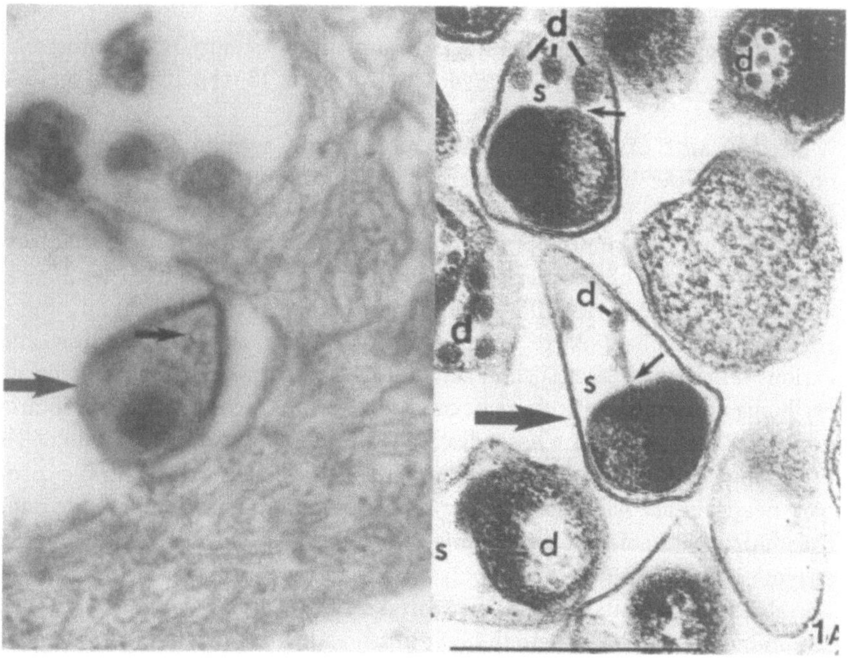

Figure 6.3. Atheroma structures compared to *Chlamydia* TWAR Pear-shaped structure of atheroma (*left red arrow*) compared to cultured TWAR organism (*right, red arrow*). Both have a similar pear shape, large periplasmic space, and minute electron-dense bodies (*black arrows*). (Electron micrograph for comparison from Chi et al. [6], with permission from the *Journal of Bacteriology*.)

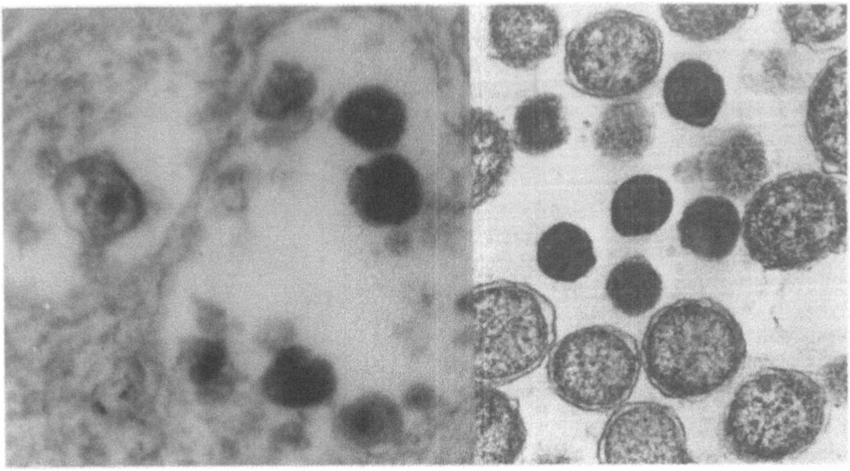

FIGURE 6.4. Atheroma structures compared to *Chlamydia* IOL 207. Atheroma structures (*left*) compared to cultured *Chlamydia pneumoniae* strain IOL 207 (*right*): both show similar small round dense structures. (Electron micrograph for comparison from Carter et al. [5], with permission from the *Journal of General Microbiology*.)

These morphological features opened up the possibility of the atheroma strain being some type of *Chlamydia* TWAR germ [5–11]. Was this feasible clinically?

Infection with *Chlamydia pneumoniae* is usually asymptomatic and causes no illness, the persons being unaware of any infection. However, the organism sometimes causes flu-like illness, pharyngitis, sinusitis, bronchitis, ear infections, community-acquired pneumonia, exacerbations of asthma, and exacerbations of chronic obstructive airway disease. There has also been serological association of the germ with a variety of other diseases such as meningoencephalitis, Guillain–Barre syndrome, myocarditis, and endocarditis, and various different diseases such as sarcoidosis, arthritis, a skin condition called erythema nodosum, cystic fibrosis, cancer of the lung, acute myocardial infarction, and chronic coronary heart disease [12]. In Finland it was found that 68% of patients with myocardial infarction and 50% of patients with chronic coronary heart disease had raised *Chlamydia* TWAR antibodies compared to controls. Also, 68% of myocardial infarction patients had sero-conversion in enzyme immunoassay with lipopolysaccharide (LPS) antigen. This response was absent in patients with chronic coronary heart disease and controls [13]. The immune complexes were thought to have an effect by activating anaphylactic products leading to inflammation, platelet aggregation, and vasospasm of coronary arteries, thus increasing the chance of myocardial infarction. Later studies found that there was a slight association of *Chlamydia pneumoniae* and ischemic heart disease, but this occurred more in smokers [14].

The majority of adults have serological evidence of past infection by this germ. Initial infection is most common in the 5- to 14-year-old age group. Serological studies indicate that it is infrequent in children under 5 years of age and increases in incidence until age 20, by which time it is found in 50% of persons. The incidence increases with age and in the elderly has a seroprevalence of 75%. As the antibody response lasts for 3 to 5 years, the suggestion is that most people are infected and reinfected throughout life. The organism has a global distribution, being more common in tropical, less-developed countries, where those younger than 5 years of age tend to be infected, which is uncommon in the United States. Serological testing of banked serum also indicates that the germ is not new but has been around at least since 1963. It is claimed humans are the only known source, although there has been a report that the germ is found in some animals.

Transmission is usually from asymptomatic carriers, and the germ is transmitted relatively inefficiently. Transmission is believed to be from person to person via respiratory secretions.

6.4. Other *Chlamydia* Species

There were descriptions of veterinary strains of *Chlamydia* that infect animals: *trachomitis* species, which infect mouse, hamster, and swine, and *psittaci* species, which infect birds, sheep, cattle, the cat family, guinea pigs, and horses. Was the atheroma germ related to a veterinary or a new human *Chlamydia* species?

At the time the closest one could come to the Chlamydia *species of atheroma was some type of* Chlamydia *TWAR or IOL207.* However, it did not seem plausible that the exact same strain of germ could be responsible for both acute pneumonia and a chronic necrotic atheroma lesion, two totally different pathological lesions.

It was necessary to try and identify this germ in atheroma, but exactly how to go about this was not all that clear.

References

1. Collier LH. *Chlamydia*. In: Topley and Wilson's principles of bacteriology, virology and immunity, 8th ed, vol 2. London: Edward Arnold, 1990:630–646.
2. Schafner W. TWAR. In: Mandel GL, Bennett JE, Dolin R (eds) Principles and practice of infectious diseases, 3rd ed. New York: Churchill Livingstone, 1990:1443–1444.
3. Saikku P, Wang SP, Kleemola M, et al. An epidemic of mild pneumonia due to an unusual strain of *Chlamydia psittaci*. J Infect Dis 1985;151(5):832–839.
4. Kuo C-C, Chen HH, Wang AP, et al. Identification of a new group of *Chlamydia psittaci* strain called TWAR. J Clin Microbiol 1986;24:1034–1037.

5. Carter MW, Al-Mahdawi SAH, Giles IG, et al. Nucleotide sequence and taxonomic value of the major outer membrane protein gene of *Chlamydia pneumoniae* IOL-207. J Gen Microbiol 1991;137:465–475.
6. Chi EY, Kuo C-C, Grayston JT. Unique ultrastructure of the elementary body of *Chlamydia* sp. TWAR. J Bacteriol 1987;169:3757–3763.
7. Kuo C-C, Chi EY, Grayston JT Ultrastructural entry of *Chlamydia* strain TWAR into He La cells. Infect Immun 1988;56(6):1668–1672.
8. Popov VL, Shatkin AA, Pankratova VN, et al. Ultrastructure of *Chlamydia pneumoniae* in cell culture. FEMS Microbiol Lett 1991;84:129–134.
9. Miyashita N, Kanemoto Y, Matsumoto A. The morphology of *Chlamydia pneumoniae*. J Med Microbiol 1993;38:418–425.
10. Wolf K, Fischer E, Hacksadt T. Ultrastructural analyses of developmental events in *Chlamydia pneumoniae*-infected cells. Infect Immun 2000;68(4):2379–2385.
11. Yang SP, Cummings PK, Patton DL, et al. Ultrastructural lung pathology of experimental *Chlamydia pneumoniae* pneumonitis in mice. J Infect Dis 1994;170:464–467.
12. Grayston JT. Infections caused by *Chlamydia pneumoniae* strain TWAR. Clin Infect Dis 1992;15:757–763.
13. Saikku P, Leinonen M, Mattila K, et al. Serological evidence of an association of a novel *Chlamydia* TWAR, with coronary artery disease and acute myocardial infarction. Lancet 1988;2:983–986.
14. Thom DH, Grayston JT, Siscovick DS, et al. Association of prior infection with *Chlamydia pneumoniae* and angiographically demonstrated coronary artery disease. JAMA 1992;268(1):68–72.

7
Identification of the Atheroma Germ

Naming the culprit

7.1. Attempts at Identification of the Germ

Now here was a major problem. *Who was going to believe the story?* There had to be some type of confirmatory evidence, and fairly convincing evidence at that, if anyone was to take the concept of atheroma containing *Chlamydia* germs seriously. Everyone accepts that the structures which make up atheroma are inert lipid droplets. They even call it a lipid-rich pool. Any suggestion of a germ would be seen as a major heretical deviation in the accepted knowledge of the disease. Introducing such a new concept is not an easy task. Not only would it be necessary to prove that the lipid of atheroma is in fact a *Chlamydia* germ, but also the exact *Chlamydia* species or strain would have to be identified. For precise identification, microbiologists rely on methods such as culture, immunocytochemistry, and genetic studies, in addition to morphology.

To try and identify the germ, culture seemed the simplest and most conclusive method. If membranous structures are fatty *Chlamydia* germs, then it should be possible to *grow these organisms* in a cell culture medium. I sent a few samples of the fatty atheroma material for possible cell culture. In retrospect, it is not surprising that no organisms were cultured. Culture is not so simple, and is highly specialized, involving different media and methods. One cannot just request culture. Also, many germs are not culturable. In fact, some *Chlamydia* are notoriously difficult organisms to culture.

There were other ways to identify the germ. New technology has opened up other methods of identification in addition to the traditional basis for identification of isolation or propagation by culture. The rapidly expanding methods, such as using part of the germ genomic material, the 16S rRNA sequences, for phylogenetic, evolutionary, and diagnostic studies, offer an opportunity for approaches to identification other than culture.

The 16 rRNA genes are found in all bacteria. Highly variable portions of the 16 rRNA sequence provide unique signatures to any bacterium. Special primers may be designed to recognize conserved gene sequences and amplify some of the diagnostic regions. The procedure has been extended to study infected mammalian tissue and avoids the need to purify the germ. This method has led to identification of previously uncharacterized pathogens in pathological lesions.

So, it appeared possible to extract and sequence extracted genetic material from a lesion, feed the information into a computer, compare this to genetic material of known germs, and so get an idea of the type of germ that is present.

However, the problem with using this method for diagnosing the atheroma germ was the extraction, sequencing, and typing of the genetic material, which is an expensive procedure in the domain of biochemistry and molecular biology. At the time, no one really believed there are germs in atheroma, and there was little enthusiasm, from these quarters, to embark on such an expensive and complicated exercise.

Why not speak to experts in the field? Perhaps there was something further that could be done to identify the germ. I thought that a talk to the microbiologists in the next building might help. Microbiologists are people who study germs and know all about germs. I walked through the gate of the microbiology institute, up to the first building on the right, then up a flight of stairs, turned left, and knocked on the door of the bacteriology department. Could I speak to the microbiologist? I introduced myself. I am a pathologist and have been looking at the fat that clogs arteries. I went through the whole story. The fat when examined with an electron microscope does not look like fat at all but looks rather like a colony or collection of millions of germs. Here are photographs of the germs. Would it be possible to identify this germ? They consist of different shapes, some round, some pear shaped, and some contain dense nuclear material and a double membrane cell wall. There are some dividing and budding forms, some larger forms, which grow in the cell cytoplasm, in vacuoles. The germs are larger than viruses but smaller than bacteria. Only two types of organisms of similar size are found in human disease: the genera *Rickettsia* and *Chlamydia*. They do not look like the elongated *Rickettsia* germs at all but could most certainly fit in with *Chlamydia*.

The microbiologists confirmed that the only *Chlamydia* germs known to occur in humans at the time were *Chlamydia trachomatis* and *Chlamydia psittaci*. One caused eye infections and sexually transmitted disease and the other caused pneumonia and was transmitted by birds. Atheroma could not be related to either of these germs. There were other *Chlamydia* species in animals, and there was a new *Chlamydia* species, TWAR, that had recently been described in humans. No one was seriously interested in doing tests to look into identification of the germ. The belief was that atheroma consisted of cholesterol and there was really no point in wasting time to show that it is a type of *Chlamydia* germ.

7.2. Positive Identification of *Chlamydia* TWAR

The species *Chlamydia* TWAR was very new, and there was no means to test for the germ at the time. Not in South Africa. Why not contact the University of Washington in Seattle, where they had described this new germ? Send some electron micrographs to the authors who had described the features of the new germ, in culture, and ask if they looked similar, and if there was some way to positively identify the germ as a type of *Chlamydia*. I sent some photographs to Professor Ted Kuo, the corresponding author, who had described the electron microscopic features of the new *Chlamydia* TWAR species, at the University of Washington. Yes, came back the reply, the electron micrographs showed structures that had some similar features to the *Chlamydia* TWAR germs, which they had described. There were questions. Where had I found the germs? If I wished I could send tissue for them to run some tests, to confirm *Chlamydia* germs were present and to try and definitely identify the *Chlamydia* species.

During the next few months I collected samples that contained these funny little creatures in the arteries, bought special containers, bought blocks of dry ice, packed the specimens in containers with dry ice, and couriered the frozen tissue samples halfway across the world, to Professor Kuo in Seattle, for further tests.

Identification was an involved process and stretched over many months. A few months down the line, I received a fax. *The message said there was exciting news.* Chlamydia *germs had been identified in the atheroma tissue that I had sent.* Further tests were going to be done to determine the exact species of *Chlamydia* in the lesions.

Another few months passed and, there was another fax. Further studies had been done to identify the germ more precisely. *The exact species of the germ in atheroma lesions was* Chlamydia *TWAR.*

So began a detailed study that lasted a year, in which time I sent more than 60 arterial specimens for testing. *At the end of the study it was established that there were germs in atheroma that looked like* Chlamydia, *contained TWAR antigens, and contained TWAR genetic material.* Was this germ only in South African atheroma lesions or did it also occur in other parts of the world?

The name of the germ was later changed to *Chlamydia pneumoniae* and subsequently to *Chlamydophila pneumoniae*. The name *Chlamydia atheroma* was not considered.

7.3. Methods of Identification

Here are some of the different methods that have been used to detect and confirm the presence of *Chlamydia pneumoniae* in atheroma.

7.3.1. Immunocytochemistry

Specific antibodies attach to specific germs. Antigen detection methods make use of TWAR antibodies labeled with a peroxidase stain for histological detection or a fluorescent marker for immunofluorescence detection. In histological sections, the peroxidase-positive antibody is seen as a dark brown stain. In immunofluorescence detection, the tissue is examined with a special microscope that shows the fluorescent stain (see Figure 7.1).

7.3.2. Polymerase Chain Reaction

Another method of diagnosis is extraction of genetic material from the specimen using the polymerase chain reaction (PCR) method. This technology can amplify very small amounts of DNA or RNA. Genetic material is extracted from atheroma and amplified. Then the products are visualized by agarose gel electrophoresis and compared to the genetic material of known *Chlamydia* germs. This method identifies the presence of *Chlamydia* genetic material.

7.3.3. Genetic Sequencing

For more detailed identification of genetic material, there are methods to clone and sequence the amplification products of the genetic material and then analyze the sequence of components. The genetic material in atheroma contains DNA products identical to those of *Chlamydia pneumoniae*.

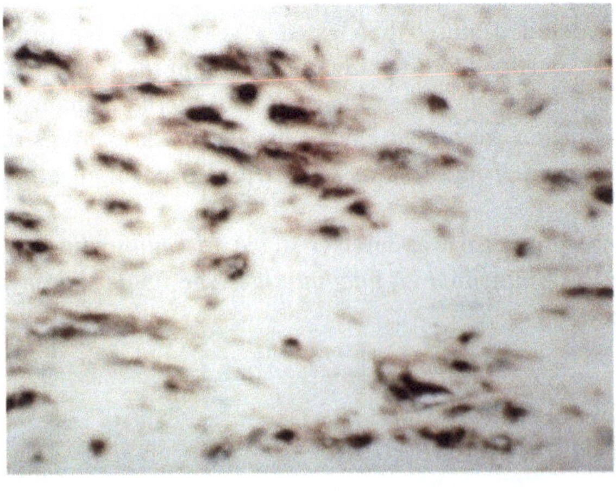

FIGURE 7.1. Immunoperoxidase stain. Atheroma showing positive immunoperoxidase staining for *Chlamydia* in some muscle cells (dark brown stain); this shows that *Chlamydia* antigens are present.

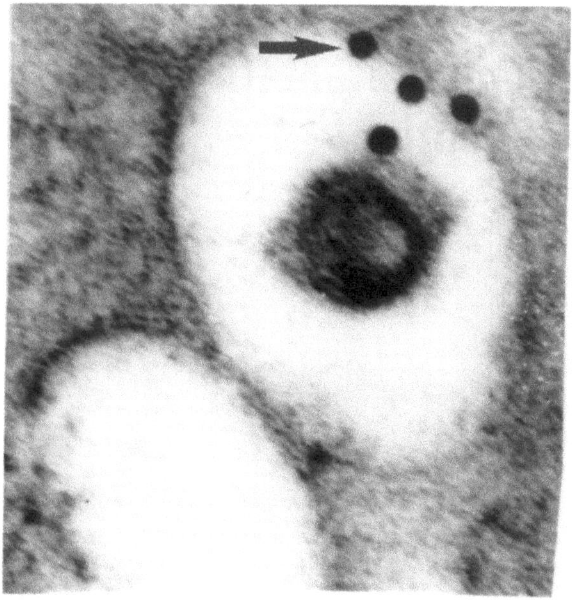

Figure 7.2. Immunogold labeling of fatty structures. Immunogold labeling shows gold beads with *Chlamydia* antibodies attached to some fatty structures in atheroma. (From Shor and Phillips [see Chapter 13: reference 6], with permission from the *Cardiovascular Journal of South Africa*.)

7.3.4. Immunogold Labeling

To definitely identify the structures as *Chlamydia* under the electron microscope, I used a procedure by which monoclonal antibodies (which specifically attach to *Chlamydia* germs) were attached to very small gold beads. Atheroma tissue was then incubated with the antibody and attached gold beads. When the tissue sections were examined under the electron microscope, it was noted that in some areas gold beads attached to lipid membranous structures, indicating these may well be *Chlamydia* organisms (see Figure 7.2).

8 Publications, Presentations, and Confirmation

8.1. Publications [1–3]

A discovery is meaningless if the findings are not published in a scientific or medical journal. Publishing in a journal is not an easy process. There are a limited number of medical journals, and the number of the many articles submitted for consideration for publication far exceeds the journal space available. It has been stated that less than 5% of articles submitted are published and more than 95% are rejected. There is just not enough space to accommodate all the articles that are submitted. On the other hand, there is tremendous pressure to publish. Publish or perish is a well-known fact. Unfortunately, a substantial amount of research just does not get published.

Publication of controversial articles is even more difficult. Suggesting that fat structures are mistaken germs is open to all kinds of ridicule by reviewers and editors, not to mention the readership.

The discovery of *Chlamydia pneumoniae* germs in atherosclerosis and fatty streak lesions was first published in the *South African Medical Journal* in 1992 [1]. Ten cases that were examined by electron microscopy and 7 which had been examined by immunocytochemistry were described. The discovery had been made toward the end of 1990, and the tests were completed in 1991. Before the original publication, the manuscript had been submitted to the *American Journal of Pathology* for review. The editor commented that the journal was open to publication of the article but would require more tests to identify the germ. The *Lancet* was not interested in the article, and submission to the journal *Arteriosclerosis and Thrombosis* had been unsuccessful.

The article was later republished in the *Year Book of Infectious Diseases* [2]. The comment of the editor was that the findings were amazing and future studies would be interesting.

A more detailed article on the demonstration of the germs in atherosclerosis lesions by Professor Kuo et al., in the *Journal of Infectious Diseases*, followed. The study consisted of an additional 36 cases of atheroma, in greater detail, and included immunocytochemistry, polymerase chain reaction (PCR) with sequencing, and culture studies [3].

8.2. Presentations [4–10]

There were presentations of the preliminary findings at congresses. For instance, in 1991 the finding was presented at an annual pathology congress. A few hours drive by car. Why not present a paper at the congress? I was a little in the dark as what to expect. Of course I thought that everyone would find that heart attacks, strokes, and other vascular problems attributable to a germ would be of some interest. At congresses there are hundreds of presentations, turned out one after the other like clockwork, the good and the bad. The presentation of *Chlamydia* germs in atheroma was just another presentation, received with some skepticism, to say the least. I did not know at the time that this skepticism was to continue in response to all the many subsequent presentations on the subject. Every presentation or lecture on the subject that atheroma did not consist of cholesterol or inert lipid, as everyone thought, but germs, a colony of *Chlamydia* germs, was usually met with some opposition. To suggest that an error of a major lesion had occurred, and that we were dying of an infection and not gluttony, cholesterol, and lifestyle, was simply against the tide of current thinking, and unacceptable as such.

The presentation of the finding of *Chlamydia* in atherosclerosis in conjunction with the University of Washington, at the 92nd Congress of Microbiology at New Orleans in 1992, elicited a fair amount of interest, and it had more credibility with the combination of detection methods that were used to show the presence of the germ. However, it was still viewed as a strange finding with questionable significance.

The arguments were always similar. Everyone knows that arteries are blocked by cholesterol because of too much fat in the blood. Atheroma consists of lipid and cholesterol. Every textbook says so.

Every group of medical or scientific personnel had their special reasons for nonacceptance. Pathologists examine tissue but not germs. Microbiologists study germs but not pathological lesions such as atheroma. Biochemists are expert in measuring the patient's cholesterol and other fats in the blood and know all about fat metabolism, but are unaware of what atheroma fat looks like, and do not study germs. Clinicians and cardiologists are expert in diagnosis and treatment, but do not examine fatty atheroma structures. Surgeons remove atheroma lesions but do not study their pathological features. There are very few persons indeed, if any at all, who have interest in going into a new controversial field of examining the ultrastructural features of atheroma lipid compared to the morphological features of cultured *Chlamydia* organisms. The idea seems too far fetched.

8.3. Confirmation [11–30]

Since the original discovery there have been a number of studies, using a variety of different methods, that have confirmed the presence of *Chlamydia pneumoniae* organisms in vascular tissue in different institutions in various parts of the world. Four studies from University of Washington all confirmed and extended the findings. One study from London also confirmed the presence of the germ in atheroma. A study in New York failed to detect the organisms.

More than 40 studies followed. Most confirmed the presence of *Chlamydia pneumoniae* germs in atheroma lesions in different parts of the world, but there were some studies at different institutions that failed to find the organisms. Questions of methodology were blamed for these discrepancies and led to attempts to try to standardize the methods of PCR and immunocytochemistry of *Chlamydia pneumoniae* detection.

Culture of the atheroma specimens that were originally sent to the University of Washington was negative. The organism is notoriously difficult to culture.

In 1996, Ramirez et al. reported the first successful isolation of *Chlamydia pneumoniae* from a coronary artery after having studied 12 explanted hearts. However, growth could only be achieved in a single case of a 56-year-old patient with severe coronary artery disease [26]. A year later, Jackson et al., studying 25 carotid endarterectomy specimens, succeeded in isolating *Chlamydia pneumoniae* from the specimen of a 60-year-old patient [27]. Maass et al. successfully cultured *Chlamydia pneumoniae* from 11 of 70 coronary endarterectomy specimens and restenotic bypass samples [28]. Apfalter et al. isolated *Chlamydia pneumoniae* from 3 of 38 atheromatous samples from aorta and femoral artery [29]. Karlsson et al. cultured *Chlamydia pneumoniae* germs from half of abdominal aortic aneurysms from a series of cases that they studied [30].

Positive culture of the organism, in a viable state in the lesion, gave added credibility to the finding that *Chlamydia* germs inhabit atheroma lesions.

8.4. Possible Special Strain of *Chlamydia pneumoniae* [31–40]

In contrast to other *Chlamydia* species, only one strain of *Chlamydia pneumoniae* is thought to exist. However, because of the unique morphological features of the germ in atheroma, and the unlikelihood of the exact same strain infecting artery and lung tissue, the finding of an unique arterial strain was always a possibility. From a medical point of view it is difficult to reconcile the fact that one germ can cause different diseases, one acute and the other chronic, one causing acute pneumonia and the other causing chronic necrosis of arteries. Germs just do not behave in that manner. Every germ causes a specific type of lesion. For instance, one strain of *Chlamydia trachomatis* causes trachoma of the eye, another strain a sexually transmitted disease, and another strain causes another disease, lymphogranuloma venereum, affecting the lymph nodes. The claim that one strain of *Chlamydia pneumoniae* is capable of causing different pathological lesions is unusual.

There is now evidence filtering through that there may be different *Chlamydia pneumoniae* strains, after all. Recent sequencing of the complete genome together with proteonomic analysis and antigenic studies indicate that different strains of *Chlamydia pneumoniae* exist and that one of these may be the arterial strain that infects arteries and causes atheroma. So here is an interesting finding. *The germ that destroys arteries may be a special unique pathogenic strain of* Chlamydia pneumoniae [31]. Even more interesting are the findings that some *Chlamydia pneumoniae* germs contain virus-like particles, called *bacteriophages* [34]. *There are suggestions that these phages (Cpn1) may confer the pathogenicity of the* Chlamydia pneumoniae *germ on vascular tissue.*

References

1. Shor A, Kuo C-C, Patton DL. Detection of *Chlamydia pneumoniae* in coronary arterial fatty streaks and atheromatous plaques. S Afr Med J 1992;82:158–161.
2. Barza MJ. Detection of *Chlamydia pneumoniae*. In: Keusch GT, Woolf SM (eds) Coronary arterial fatty streaks and atheromatous plaques. Year book of infectious diseases. St. Louis: Mosby, 1994:365–367.
3. Kuo C-C, Shor A, Campbell LA, et al. Demonstration of *Chlamydia pneumoniae* in atherosclerotic lesions of coronary arteries. J Infect Dis 1993;167:841–849.
4. Shor A, Brunton JG, Van Sittert GCH. Preliminary study of structures found in human coronary artery lesions. Electron Microscopic Society of South Africa, Cape Town, December 1991, pp 241–242.
5. Shor A. *Chlamydia* TWAR in coronary atheroma: an ultrastructural study. Presented at 31st Annual Congress of Society of Pathology of South Africa, 30 June to 3 July, 1991, Warmbaths, South Africa.
6. Shor A, Kuo C-C, Patton DL, et al. Detection of *Chlamydia pneumoniae* in coronary atheroma plaque. Presented at 92nd American Society of Microbiology Meeting, 26–30 May, 1992, New Orleans, LA, USA.
7. Shor A, Pantanowitz D, Veller M, et al. New avenues of research in *Chlamydia* related atheroma. Presented at 20th Biennial Congress of Southern Africa, 31 August–5 September, 1996, Victoria Falls, Zimbabwe.
8. Shor A. Treatment of chlamydial atherosclerotic lesions. In: Abstracts of 2nd International Meeting of Interventional Cardiology, Jerusalem, Israel, June–July 1997. J Invas Cardiol 1997;9(suppl C).
9. Shor A, Pantanowitz D, Veller M. The current status of the association between *Chlamydia pneumoniae* and atherosclerosis. Presented to the Vascular Society of Southern Africa, Sun City, 1–4 August, 1999.
10. Shor A. Atherosclerosis: role of *Chlamydia pneumoniae* in atherogenesis and lipid production. Presented at LASSA Congress, 2–7 April, 2000, Durban, South Africa.
11. Camm AJ, Grayston JT. *Chlamydia pneumoniae* in the cardiovascular system. Atherosclerosis (Suppl) 1998;140:S1–S35.
12. Campbell LA, Kuo C-C, Grayston JT. *Chlamydia pneumoniae* and cardiovascular disease. Emerg Infect Dis 1998;l4(4):571–579.

13. Gaydos CA. *Chlamydia pneumoniae*: a review and evidence in coronary artery disease. Clin Microbiol Newsl 1995;17(7):49–54.
14. Grayston JT, Kuo C-C, Campbell LA, et al. *Chlamydia pneumoniae* strain TWAR and atherosclerosis. Eur Heart J 1993;14(suppl K):66–71.
15. Grayston JT. *Chlamydia* in atherosclerosis. Circulation 1993;87(4):1408–1409.
16. Grayston JT. Does *Chlamydia pneumoniae* cause atherosclerosis? Arch Surg 1999;134:930–934.
17. Ewald PW, Cochran GM. *Chlamydia pneumoniae* and cardiovascular disease: an evolutionary perspective on infection and antibiotic treatment. J Infect Dis (Suppl) 2000;181(30):S394–S401.
18. Taylor-Robinson D. *Chlamydia pneumoniae* in vascular tissue. Atherosclerosis 1998;140(suppl 1):s21–s24.
19. Taylor-Robinson D, Thomas BJ. *Chlamydia pneumoniae* in arteries: the facts, their interpretation, and future studies. J Clin Pathol 1998;51:793–797.
20. Quinn CT. Does *Chlamydia pneumoniae* cause coronary heart disease? Curr Opin Infect Dis 1998;11:301–307.
21. Veller M, Shor A. The role of *Chlamydia pneumoniae* in the pathogenesis of atherosclerosis. Eur J Endovasc Surg 1998;16:459–461.
22. Kuo C-C, Campbell LA. Is infection with *Chlamydia pneumoniae* a causative agent in atherosclerosis? Mol Med Today 1998;4:426–430.
23. Muhlestein JB. The link between *Chlamydia pneumoniae* and atherosclerosis. Infect Med 1997;14(5):380–382.
24. Zeeman K, Pospisil L, Canderle J, et al Direct and indirect evidence of *Chlamydia pneumoniae* in patients with significant stenosis of a carotis of atherosclerotic origin. Scripta Med (BRNO) 2004;77(3):173–180.
25. Rose AG. *Chlamydia pneumoniae* and atherosclerosis. (Editorial.) Cardiovasc J S Afr 2000;11(1):11–12.
26. Ramirez JA and the *Chlamydia pneumoniae*/Atherosclerosis Study Group. Isolation of *Chlamydia pneumoniae* from the coronary artery of a patient with coronary atherosclerosis. Ann Intern Med 1996;125:979–982.
27. Jackson LA, Campbell LA, Kuo C-C, et al. Isolation of *Chlamydia pneumoniae* from a carotid endarterectomy specimen. J Infect Dis 1997;176(19):292–295.
28. Maass M, Bartels C, Engel PM, et al. Endovascular presence of viable *Chlamydia pneumoniae* is a common phenomenon in coronary artery disease. J Am Coll Cardiol 1998;31:827–832.
29. Apfalter P, Loidl M, Nadrchal R, et al. Isolation and continuous growth of *Chlamydia pneumoniae* from arterectomy specimens. Eur J Clin Microbiol Infect Dis 2000; 19:305–308.
30. Karlsson L, Gnarpe J, Naas J, et al. Detection of viable *Chlamydia pneumoniae* in abdominal aortic aneurysms. Eur J Vasc Endovasc Surg 2000;19(6):630–635.
31. Gieffers J, Durling L, Ouellette SP, et al. Genotypic differences in the *Chlamydia pneumoniae* tyr P gene related to vascular tropism and pathogenicity. J Infect Dis 2003;188(8):1085–1093.
32. Jantos CA, Heck S, Roggendorf R, et al. Antigenic and molecular analyses of different *Chlamydia pneumoniae* strains. J Clin Microbiol 1997;35(3):620–623.
33. Kalman S, Mitchell W, Marathe R, et al. Comparative genomes of *Chlamydia pneumoniae* and *C. trachomatis*. Nat Genet 1999;21:385–389.
34. Karunakaran KP, Blanchard JF, Raudonikiene A, et al. Molecular and seroepidemiology of *Chlamydia pneumoniae* bacteriophage (Cpn1). J Clin Microbiol 2002;40(11): 4010–4014.

35. Kutlin A, Flegg C, Stenzel D, et al. Ultrastructural study of *Chlamydia pneumoniae* in a continuous model. J Clin Microbiol 2001;39:3721–3723.
36. Molestina RE, Dean D, Miller RD, et al. Characterisation of a strain of *Chlamydia pneumoniae* isolated from a coronary atheroma by analyses of the Omp 1 gene and biological activity in human endothelial cells. Infect Immun 1998;66(4):1370–1376.
37. Osserwaarde JM, Meijer A. Molecular evidence for existence of additional members of order *Chlamydiales*. Microbiology 1999;145(pt 2):411–417.
38. Read TD, Brunham RC, Shen SR, et al. Genome sequences of *Chlamydia trachomatis* MoPn and *Chlamydia pneumoniae* AR39. Nucleic Acids Res 2000;25:1397–1406.
39. Shirai M, Hirakawa H, Kimoto M, et al. Comparison of whole genome sequence of *Chlamydia pneumoniae* J138 from Japan and CWL029 from U.S.A. Nucleic Acids Res 2000;28:2311–2314.
40. Everett KD, Bush RM, Andersen AA. Amended description of the order Chlamydiales, proposal of Parachlamydiaceae fam. nov. and Simkaniaceae fam. nov. containing one monocytic genus, revised taxonomy of the family Chlamydiaceae, including a new genus and five new species, and standards for the identification of organisms. Int J Syst Bacteriol 1999;49(pt 2):415–440.

9
Chlamydia Are Inherent Components of Atheroma

Do all lesions contain Chlamydia germs?

Positivity rates for finding *Chlamydia pneumoniae* germs in atheroma depending on the methods used for detection vary from 0% to 100% (mean, 60%), with a few studies failing to detect the organisms by polymerase chain reaction (PCR). The many reviews on the subject of detection indicate increasing acceptance of the presence of *Chlamydia* organisms in human atherosclerotic lesions, but there are suggestions for a need to improve and standardize the diagnostic techniques.

9.1. Serology Not Helpful

Seroepidemiological surveys may offer some information on heart disease but unfortunately are unable to determine which patients have *Chlamydia* in their arteries. Serology usually does not indicate when infection occurs or its spatial relationship to commencement of atherosclerosis. To assess the relationship with atheroma, one would have to assess the degree of atheroma in each patient. Since the first study in Finland by Saikku et al. of antibody titers in patients with coronary artery disease and myocardial infarction, there have been more than 100 papers attempting to show an association between patients who suffer ischemic heart diseases, or strokes, and antibody titers to *Chlamydia pneumoniae*. Results have varied. Studies are concerned with different populations, use different criteria for cases, are sometimes not adjusted for potential confounders such as cigarette smoking, and are consequently prone to different biases. There have been meta-analyses of the various studies [1–3]. Danesh et al. published the results of a large population based prospective study with a meta-analysis of 14 prospective published studies [1]. The studies included a total of 3169 cases. The studies overall did not generally support an association of *Chlamydia pneumoniae* antibodies and cardiovascular disease. It should be pointed out that with the high prevalence of antibody in middle and old age and therefore in control populations, there is reduced opportunity to show a difference in the frequency of antibody in cases versus controls. There is little evidence that seroepidemiological studies can separate those with prior infection from those with chronic infection. Antibody status is not always in tandem with the severity of *Chlamydia* infection, and studies are not designed to examine the presence of germs in atheromatous lesions [4].

9.2. Previous Journal Articles on Atheroma Contain Pictures of Unrecognized *Chlamydia* Germs

There are, however, reasons to believe that *Chlamydia pneumoniae* germs are inherent components of atheroma lesions.

As pointed out, the central lipid-rich core of atheroma consists largely of structures called membrane-bound fatty structures, lipid droplets, vesicles, dense bodies, and unknown bodies. Pathology journals illustrate these different types of structures, considered to be altered lipid [see Chapter 5: references 1–11]. *However, many of these fatty structures resemble cultured* Chlamydia *germs, as illustrated in microbiology journals and textbooks* [see Chapter 5: references 12–23]. This finding implies that *Chlamydia*-like structures are common and inherent components of atheroma gruel, at least since 1961, when the first electron micrographs of these structures were illustrated.

Why has the germ gone unnoticed for so long? One reason is that anatomical pathologists were not microbiologists, and microbiologists certainly did not study the morphological features of fat droplets in atheroma. The germs were simply not recognized as such and were accepted as strange-looking lipid droplets.

The other problem is that, before the mid-1980s, even if it was considered that the lipid structures in atheroma were *Chlamydia* germs, it would not have been possible to identify them, as such. The only *Chlamydia* species known at the time were the trachoma- and psittacosis-type agents. Detection studies for both these *Chlamydia* agents in atheroma would have proven to be negative. Since then, a number of new *Chlamydia* species have been identified. It was only after 1986, following identification of the new *Chlamydia* TWAR species and development of PCR and immunocytochemical technology for identification, that it became possible for the germ to be identified in atheroma lesions.

An article published in 1945 associated the virus of lymphogranuloma venereum (today known as *Chlamydia trachomatis*) with arteriosclerosis of the arteries, and also other vascular conditions such as Buerger's disease, giant cell arteritis , temporal arteritis, and periarteritis. The article was based on an observation that scarring and fibrosis caused by this organism may be similar to the scarring and fibrosis that take place in arteries [5]. Could this in some way be taken as an inkling that the *Chlamydia* germ had in the past, somewhere along the line, somehow been considered to play a role in atherosclerosis? Hardly. The lesion of atherosclerosis was not mentioned, *Chlamydia* germs as we know them today were not yet discovered, and certainly the lymphogranuloma venereum germ is not present in atheroma.

9.3. Persons with Congenital Raised Cholesterol Contain *Chlamydia pneumoniae* Germs in Atheroma [6–10]

There is another reason to suspect that *Chlamydia pneumoniae* germs are prevalent in atheroma lesions.

Homozygous familial hypercholesterolemia (HFH) is a genetic disease in which children inherit the disorder of high serum cholesterol from both parents. Babies who are born with this disease are characterized by markedly elevated levels of plasma cholesterol. If untreated, the majority of patients with this disorder die of accelerated atherosclerosis before the age of 30 years [6]. The association of hypercholesterolemia and premature severe atherosclerosis in this disease forms the strongest basis on which cholesterol is implicated in atheroma. The condition affects only 1 in 1 million persons and, because of the rarity of the condition, the pathology has only been studied in a few cases [7,8]. Examination of these atheroma lesions is invaluable to understanding the link between raised cholesterol and atherosclerosis. Studies have described the atherosclerotic lesion in this condition as similar to the conventional fibronecrotic human atheroma lesion [7], but another study of a lesion has suggested that there are differences [8]. One would expect that this lesion must surely be caused by fat infiltration and therefore be a different lesion from that which clogs the arteries because of *Chlamydia* germs.

There were 26 cases being treated for this disease in the lipid clinic at the University hospital. It was really important to have a good look at the atheroma lesions in these cases. One case was an 11-year-old HFH who had died of a heart attack, but the parents refused to allow an autopsy to be performed on the child. Another case was a 16-year-old girl who died suddenly in a swimming pool. An autopsy was performed to establish the cause of death. We obtained special written permission from her parents, as required by law at that time, to specially examine the arteries of this patient.

The patient was a 16-year-old female HFH, confirmed on DNA analysis of the LDL receptor gene. She had been on high doses of lipid-lowering drug therapy since the age of 7 years, but despite this her serum cholesterol level could not be reduced below 10 mmol/L. Before her death, *Chlamydia pneumoniae* serology showed an IgG titer of 1/128. In other words, she had come into contact with *Chlamydia pneumoniae* germs.

At autopsy, it was ascertained that the child had indeed died of a heart attack. The salient features were marked and severe atheroma of all the arteries. The main artery of the body, the aorta, and arteries to the heart or coronary arteries, arteries to the brain, and also the lung arteries and pulmonary arteries, were all involved Atheroma had blocked the arteries to the heart muscle, and the heart showed an infarct, an area of dead heart muscle, to be more precise. She had suffered a heart attack, and this had resulted in her death [9,10].

Microscopy of the atheroma showed both early and quite advanced lesions, and a large number of *Chlamydia* inclusion bodies were noted to be present.

Electron microscopy showed Chlamydia pneumoniae-*like structures present in the cells and in the central fatty atheroma area.*

Immunoperoxidase staining was positive for Chlamydia pneumoniae using monoclonal antibody M660 (Dako).

Polymerase chain reaction testing was positive for Chlamydia pneumoniae germs.

Everyone believes that the blockage is caused by high cholesterol, which infiltrates and blocks the artery. Now here was something really strange. Even in people with very high cholesterol, the atheroma lesion still contains the same *Chlamydia* germ, same as in everyone else [9,10].

There must obviously be some tie between cholesterol and infection with the germ; otherwise, why should the HFH patients develop such severe *Chlamydia* infection and atheroma at such an early age? Here was a new challenge. Explain how high cholesterol causes *Chlamydia pneumoniae* infection.

The primary defect of HFH is the lack of cholesterol cell receptors. The cells are incapable of taking up cholesterol. Because of this, the blood cholesterol is raised. Raised serum cholesterol is therefore a secondary phenomenon of the disease. The first thing that had to determined, and is still not clear, is whether the problem is caused by the primary defect of the disease, which is being born without cholesterol cell receptors, or whether the resultant raised blood cholesterol is the culprit. Without cholesterol receptors, cells cannot take up and utilize the cholesterol. It has recently been found that if the body does not have enough cholesterol, all kinds of cellular functions are compromised. The defense mechanisms and other mechanisms become ineffective. This may be the problem.

On the other hand, the germ needs cholesterol to grow and flourish, to build cell walls and vacuoles in which to live. Of particular interest in this regard are the recent findings that *Chlamydia* use cholesterol to enter and infect cells. Also, cholesterol is diverted by the cell and is used for production of the vacuole in which the germ survives. The markedly elevated serum cholesterol levels found in HFH subjects may provide a milieu for the rapid growth of *Chlamydia* organisms, leading to the rapid development, or acceleration, of atherosclerosis. In some animal models, the atherogenic effect of *Chlamydia* appears dependent on serum cholesterol levels.

The finding of *Chlamydia pneumoniae* in a patient with HFH adds further strength to the fact that *Chlamydia* germs are inherent components of atheroma lesions.

9.4. Are There Other Germs in Atheroma? [11–15]

Since the suggestion that there may be increased *Chlamydia pneumoniae* antibodies in patients who have suffered heart attacks, a number of articles have appeared in the literature showing that antibodies to multiple organisms can be associated with heart disease in the same way.

These studies examine the incidence of antibodies to various germs in heart attack patients as compared to non-heart attack patients. If there is an increased incidence of antibodies to a germ in heart attack patients, then the germs are canvassed as playing a role in causing heart attacks. An ever-increasing number of infective agents have been associated with heart attacks in this manner: cytomegalovirus, herpesvirus, *Helicobacter pylori*, dental infections, enterobacterial infections, hepatitis A, and many others.

These types of studies have raised questions as to the status of the various germs, such as bacteria, viruses, and fungal and parasitic infections in heart attack patients. Can we conclude that the studies showing previous infection by an organism has significance in the pathogenesis of later heart attacks? Conversely, can one assume that, if a person has decreased antibodies to a germ, this prevents future heart attacks?

As far as the atherosclerosis lesion is concerned, the coronary arteries contain only a small part of the atherosclerosis that is present in the arterial system and as such does not indicate the extent of the total atheroma in the vasculature. It is not correct to accept that the clinical symptom of decreased blood supply of the coronary arteries alone is an indication of the extent and severity of atherosclerotic disease. Showing that slightly more people with heart attacks have been exposed to infective organisms, sometime in their lives, is far from proving that these germs are the cause of fatty pultaceous material in arteries.

Then there are studies that look for remnants of various organisms in atheroma lesions [13,14]. In the 1980s, different types of herpes viral remnants were found in atherosclerotic lesions in the aorta and also in normal aortic tissue. Recently it has been reported that genetic material of *Helicobacter pylori*, the germ that causes stomach ulcers, and certain dental bacteria are present in atherosclerotic lesions. The finding of positive genetic material has not always been consistent; this is one of the problems encountered with use of this method of detection. Certainly complete organisms have not been shown, and it seems improbable that pathologists examining these lesions could overlook such large organisms as *Helicobacter* or dental bacteria. There is also the question as to the location of the genetic material. Is the material in the intima (where atherosclerosis occurs), or in the media or adventitia where there is no atheroma? Is the genetic material in the blood? Blood is invariably present in arterial specimens. Arteries are not only in contact with blood, but are also supplied by the vaso vasorum, which contain blood. None of these organisms has been shown to be viable. The implications of finding DNA remnants have not been fully addressed, but the question remains as to whether they could in some way produce an arterial lesion.

In animal models, different types of infectious agents have been used to produce lesions in arteries. As an example, Marek's chicken virus produces arterial lesions in chickens [15]. However, animal lesions produced by different germs experimentally have pathological features that differ from those which occur in the human atheroma lesion.

As far as human arterial lesions go, other than syphilitic aortitis, which is seldom seen today, and the very rare tuberculosis lesion, there are really no infective chronic arterial lesions described. Herpes, *Helicobacter*, dental infection, enterobacteria, and hepatitis lesions have never been described in human arteries.

References

1. Danesh J, Whincup P, Walker M, et al. *Chlamydia pneumoniae* IgG titres and coronary heart disease: prospective study and meta-analysis. BMJ 2000;321:208–212.
2. Bloemenkamp DG, Mali WP, Visseren FL. Meta-analysis of sero-epidemiological studies of the relation between *Chlamydia pneumoniae* and atherosclerosis: does study design influence results? Am Heart J 2003;145(3):409–417.
3. Wald NJ, Law MR, Morris JK, et al. *Chlamydia pneumoniae* infection and mortality from ischaemic heart disease: large prospective study. BMJ 2000;321:204–207.
4. Puolakkainen M, Kuo C-C, Shor A, et al. Serological response to *Chlamydia pneumoniae* in adults with coronary arterial fatty streaks and fibrolipid plaques. J Clin Microbiol 1993;31(8):2212–2214.
5. Coutts WE, Davila M. Lymphogranuloma venereum as a possible cause of arteriosclerosis and other arterial conditions. J Trop Med Hyg 1945;48:46–51.
6. Goldstein JL, Hobbs HH, Brown MS. Familial hypercholesterolaemia. In: Scriver CR, Beaudet AL, Sly WS, Valle D (eds) Metabolic and molecular basis of inherited disease, 7th ed. New York: McGraw-Hill 1995:1981–2030.
7. Sprecher DL, Schaefer EJ, Kent KM, et al. Cardiovascular features of homozygous familial hypercholesterolaemia: analysis of 16 patients. Am J Cardiol 1984;54:20–30.
8. Stehbens WE, Martin M. Case report. The vascular pathology of familial hypercholesterolaemia. Pathology 1991;23:1–54.
9. Shor A. Atherosclerotic lesions in a homozygous familial hypercholesterolaemic patient contains *Chlamydia pneumoniae* organisms. In: Lewis B, Halon DA, Flugelman MY, Hradec J (eds) Textbook on 4th international congress on coronary artery disease. Bologna, Italy: Monduzzi, 2000:227–230.
10. Shor A. Atherosclerosis lipid infiltration or *Chlamydia pneumoniae* infection. Circulation 2002;106(18)135e.
11. Melnick JL, Adam E, De Bakey ME. Possible role of cytomegalovirus in atherogenesis. JAMA 1990;263:2204–2207.
12. Mattila KJ, Valtonen VV, Niemenin MS, et al. Role of infection as a risk factor for atherosclerosis, myocardial infection and stroke. Clin Infect Dis 1998;26:719–734.
13. Farsak B, Yildirir A, Akyon Y, et al. Detection of *Chlamydia pneumoniae* and *Helicobacter pylori* DNA in human atherosclerotic plaques by PCR. J Clin Microbiol 2000;12(38):4408–4411.
14. Haraszthy VI, Zambon JJ, Trevisan M, et al. Identification of periodontal pathogens in atheromatous plaques. Periodontology 2000;71(10)1554–1560.
15. Moss NS, Benditt EP. The ultrastructure of spontaneous and experimentally induced arterial lesions. Lab Invest 1970;25(3):231–245.

10
Do *Chlamydia* Germs Cause Atherosclerosis?

How can we determine if a germ causes a lesion?

10.1. Determining Causality

The first part of the story concerns the discovery of *Chlamydia* in atheroma. Actually, to be more precise, the discovery that many of the fat structures in atheroma are overlooked *Chlamydia* germs. We now have to examine another aspect: whether this germ is the actual cause of the atheroma lesion.

The attitude and how the scientific community views a discovery is all important. All cases in which new germs have been found in lesions have usually brought about controversy and discussion, centered around determination of significance and the possible role of the germ in lesion formation. There are conflicting ideas as how to ascertain the significance of microorganisms in a disease process. Proof of a germ being the cause of a lesion has been the greatest stumbling block to discovery in most cases.

Finding *Chlamydia* germs in atheroma lesions has been no exception. In fact, there has been some heated debate on the question of the precise role of this small creature in the atherogenic process.

There is not really a problem today with acceptance that *Chlamydia pneumoniae* organisms are present in human atheroma lesions. After all, they have been visualized specifically in these lesions, and not in normal arteries. They have also been firmly and conclusively tied to the scene of the crime. Photographed, in the vicinity of arterial damage. Their antigens have been detected, and their genetic material has been found lying around. We know the fellow is alive and well. Some of the creatures have been captured in the lesion and nourished and grown in cell culture. In fact, they have thrived and multiplied in this environment. All these aspects show *Chlamydia pneumoniae* germs are living in atheroma lesions.

But finding a germ in a lesion, or at the scene of a crime, does not always imply that the germ is definitely the cause of the damage. The germ just happen to be at the scene, at the time, a coincidence. It plays no role in the disease whatsoever. Others suggest that *Chlamydia* play some role but that it has accomplices and as such should not be held solely responsible for the crime. Then there are those who believe that this minute creature is the sole perpetrator, and should be brought to book and held personally liable for malicious damage to arteries and the formation of the lesion.

For determination of causality there are certain criteria requirements, but these are not absolute, and are based largely on probability. Because of this, there is lack of agreement in the scientific community as to the precise role of the germ in the lesion. For instance, Taylor-Robinson points out that ascertaining what is cause and what is effect, in this particular case, is much like the question of what comes first, "the chicken or the egg" [1]. Not so easy to resolve. Thomas Grayston has addressed the question as to what is needed to prove that the germ does, or does not, play a causal role in atherosclerosis. He suggests that there is no one experiment that will definitely prove or disprove the hypothesis of an etiological role for *Chlamydia pneumoniae* in atherosclerosis. Rather, a gradual accumulation of data from many investigators will lead to acceptance or rejection of the hypothesis. Proof will not be absolute but rather an overwhelming consensus of opinion by knowledgeable scientists [2].

In legal circles, murder and other crimes are investigated, evidence is accumulated, then criminals are arrested and tried in a court of law. The evidence is presented and considered by a jury or judge, a verdict is handed down, and sentence is passed. The accused is found to be either guilty or not guilty and labeled as such. In the scientific community, things are a little different. Germs or other suspects of causing a disease or lesion to humans are not arrested. The scientific and medical fraternity are not trained legal persons; there is no presentation of evidence at a trial, no court cases, no judges, and no juries. Determination as to whether a germ is responsible for a disease, or not, is by other means. Scientific methods, they are called.

10.2. Statistical Criteria

For determination of causality, microbiologists rely on statistical probabilities and fulfilment of certain criteria. One of the methods used is fulfilment of criteria as proposed by Sir Brandford Hill [3,4]. There has to be fulfilment of certain parameters such as strength, consistency, specificity, temporality, plausibility coherence, analogy, and experimental evidence in the association between germ and disease.

If one considers these factors in relation to *Chlamydia pneumoniae* organisms and atherosclerosis, there is a strong and consistent association of *Chlamydia pneumoniae* and human atherosclerotic lesions, in that the germs are found in the lesion in the majority of cases. The germs are specific to atheromatous lesions in that they are only visible and constantly found in the lesion, and not in normal arterial tissue. Germs are noted in atheromatous lesions in all major arteries, that is, aorta, coronary arteries, carotid arteries, and iliac, femoral, and pulmonary arteries. To fulfill the criteria of temporality, the organism must be found in the earliest lesion. Germs have been found in the earliest lesions in young persons and teenagers. The concept of a *Chlamydia* arterial lesion is plausible and coherent in that this particular germ is a lipophilic pathogenic organism and as such is a candidate for causing a lesion with fatty content such as atherosclerosis. *Chlamydia pneumoniae* is one of the agents that have been proposed as causing initiation of damage, in the response to injury theory of atherosclerosis, a popular theory of the atherogenic mechanism. An analogy can be drawn between atherosclerosis and other types of *Chlamydia*-related lesions such as trachoma and lymphogranuloma venereum, both of which are similar fibrotic and necrotic lesions. There are an increasing number of molecular biological studies showing that the C-reactive protein, adhesion molecules, interleukin-6, and heat shock proteins that are found in the lesion are related to the organism. Experimentally, *Chlamydia pneumoniae* germs have been cultured in aortic smooth muscle cells, endothelial cells, and macrophages, all components of atherosclerotic lesions in humans. *Chlamydia pneumoniae* arterial lesions have been produced in various animals, and a study has suggested that these lesions are preventable in animals by giving the antichlamydial agent azithromycin.

10.3. Koch's Postulates

Koch, who discovered the cause of tuberculosis, found a solution to the problem of causality. He claimed that, to prove a germ is the cause of a particular lesion, it is necessary to show that inoculation of the specific germ produces a lesion in an animal. This should then be followed by isolation of the germ from the particular lesion. Third, reinoculation of the germ isolate in another similar animal should produce the same type of lesion. Mice and rabbits have been inoculated with *Chlamydia pneumoniae* and a type of atherosclerotic lesion is produced. These lesions contain *Chlamydia pneumoniae* remnants; however, as yet it has not been possible to isolate the *Chlamydia* from these lesions and therefore reinoculate another animal [5].

10.4. Does Eradication of Germ Prove Causality?

Then there are persons who say that, to prove causality, it must be shown that eradication of the germ results in healing of the lesion. Animal studies indicate improvement of lesion. Antibiotic clinical studies have been done but these do not look at the lesion per se. As pointed out, a definitive demonstration of *Chlamydia* as the cause of atherosclerosis could result from the use of an effective vaccine in childhood. If the vaccine were widely used in a population and atherosclerosis was virtually eliminated, the hypothesis would be proven. However, it would take 40 to 50 years for definite proof. It is hardly practical to wait so long for an answer.

10.5. No Disease Without Causal Agent

Stehbens wrote an article on causality [see Chapter 3: reference 36]. He states that if an agent is the cause, it follows that without that specific agent the lesion cannot occur. He goes on to state that misuse of the word "cause" in epidemiology has wider implications, especially in a chronic disease such as atherosclerosis. Lack of differentiation of the roles of causal and associated factors can delay the concentrated effort required to seek and identify the essential cause. Upgrading the importance of noncausative factors downgrades the true cause, which is masked by a host of risk factors of less importance and dubious significance [see Chapter 3: reference 36]. This is the case with atheroma. With the hundreds of factors implicated in the disease, no one has seriously considered the extent of *Chlamydia pneumoniae* organisms in the lesion. The fact that the lesion actually consists almost exclusively of a colony of *Chlamydia* organisms is lost in a web of associated factors, risk factors, cofactors, additional factors, and statistical aspects.

Debating and considering all the foregoing factors have not resulted in a conclusion on the matter. Perhaps we should change the general question that has been posed from "Do *Chlamydia* germs fulfill requirements for causality?" to "*Have we overlooked a pathological entity, an arterial atherosclerotic* Chlamydia *lesion*?"

References

1. Taylor-Robinson D. *Chlamydia pneumoniae* in arteries: a tale of the unexpected. J Infect 1997;35:97–98.
2. Grayston JT. What is needed to prove that *Chlamydia pneumoniae* does or does not play an etiological role in atherosclerosis. J Infect Dis 2000;181:S585–S586.
3. Grayston JT. *Chlamydia pneumoniae* TWAR and atherosclerosis. In: Orfila J, Byrne GI, Chernesky M, et al. (eds) Chlamydial infections. Proceedings of the eighth international symposium of human chlamydial infections. Bolognia, Italy: Societa Editrice Esculapio, 1994:199–208.
4. Shor A, Philips JI, Ong G, et al. *Chlamydia pneumoniae* in atheroma: consideration of criteria for causality. J Clin Pathol 1998;51:812–817.
5. Fredericks DN, Relman DA. Sequence-based identification of microbial pathogens: a reconsideration of Koch's postulates. Clin Microbiol Rev 1996;9(1):18–33.

11
Pathological Lesion Diagnosis

How to determine the nature of a lesion

In all disease processes, different aspects are stressed by the microbiologist, biochemist, geneticist, statistician, clinician, etc. But it is the *specific function of the pathologist to diagnose tissue samples and lesions*. Use is made of different tools to come to some conclusion as to the nature and cause of lesions.

11.1. Lesion Examination [1–3]

Of all techniques, observation and interpretation of the pathological features are of paramount importance. There are some lesions that can be recognized by examination with the naked eye alone. Interpretation of the size, shape, color, localization, infiltration, and consistency is sometimes sufficient.

Most lesions, however, require additional microscopic examination for a diagnosis to be reached. The light microscope came into being in the seventeenth century, and soon became a tool for use in examination of tissue and cells in greater detail. This instrument remains the cornerstone for diagnosis used by the anatomical pathologist. Selected small pieces of tissue are sampled, the localization of which are documented by means of drawings or photographs. The tissue is then processed, embedded in wax blocks, cut, and stained. Sometimes special stains are used to glean more information about the tissue components. The stained slides are then examined microscopically. An image produced by a light microscope is called a light micrograph.

For greater magnification of tissue, an electron microscope is used. The images are called electron micrographs. A transmission electron micrograph is capable of showing fine cellular detail and internal structures of cells and germs in two dimensions.

The scanning electron microscope uses electrons that bounce off tissue and produce a three-dimensional view of the surface details.

Fine-needle aspirate with cytopathological examination, polymerase chain reaction (PCR) with extraction of nucleic acids, and in situ hybridization are recent developments that have helped with the study, interpretation, and diagnosis of lesions.

11.2. Lesion Diagnosis

The picture that is seen under the microscope, the architectural arrangement of cells with cytological features, and changes in connective tissue elements together with different special and immunocytochemical stains and other techniques, are all assessed and interpreted, and thus diagnosis of a lesion is reached.

Diagnosis necessitates a consideration of the multiple factors involved in the formation and pathogenesis of a disease process. Causal agents, such as microorganisms, chemicals, physical forces, genetic predisposition, and metabolic diseases, all vary in their capacity to injure tissue, and each causes specific types of injury and specific lesions. All individuals may not respond in the same way or intensity to the same agent, and the pathological processes of inflammation and immunoreactivity that occur in response to these agents do not always respond uniformly or sequentially in each individual. Some diseases produce great exaggerations of the spectrum of structural and functional cell responses compared to those that are considered normal, whereas others produce minimal subtle changes. The time involved in development of lesions is also important. Acute or sudden processes may differ greatly from their chronic or slowly occurring (over a long time) counterparts. Sometimes there is a mixture of acute processes superimposed on chronic lesions. Also, similar pathological processes may cause different changes and symptoms in different organs. One of the most misleading aspect of examination of pathological specimens involves the multiplicity of causation. Sometimes there is superimposition of one or more agents. These agents must be differentiated and the dominant causal factor of the lesion determined.

Very important decisions are based on interpretation of lesions, and pathologists will go to fairly great lengths to make a diagnosis. Surgical operations with removal of tissue or organs and even amputations of limbs, as well as implementation of treatment, chemotherapy, and radiotherapy, and sometimes life-and-death decisions, are based solely on pathological diagnosis.

11.3. Inability to Diagnose Atheroma Lesion

However, strange it may seem, with all the advanced investigative tools available today, *pathologists are still at a loss to produce a diagnosis of this necrotic lesion*. Call it what you want, pultaceous, grumous, necrotic, fatty, inflammatory. There is still no unanimity of opinion as to what it is and from where it comes.

Neville Woolf points out that in the study of atherosclerosis, as indeed in the study of all disease, the aim of the pathologist should be to delineate as accurately as possible not only the characteristic lesion, but all the pathogenic steps that delineate their base. Unfortunately, the various mechanisms playing a role in the initiation and progression of the atherosclerotic lesion are still not fully elucidated. No specific features have been documented to help make a diagnosis, and no conclusion as to the precise cause of the lesion has come forward [see Chapter 3: reference 8].

There remains a general feeling that it is old fashioned and superfluous to reexamine atherosclerosis lesions and redocument the existing features.

References

1. Cheville NF. Introduction. In: Cheville NF (ed) Cell pathology. Ames: Iowa State University Press, 1976:3–6.
2. Rosai J. Introduction. In: Rosai F (ed) Rosai and Ackerman's surgical pathology, 9th ed, vol 1. London: Elsevier, 2004:1–32.
3. Smith CJ, Scott SM, Wagner BM. The necessary role of the autopsy in cardiovascular epidemiology. Hum Pathol 1998;29(12):1469–1479.

12 Study of Atheroma Lesions

A special look at how to go about diagnosing the atheroma lesion

12.1. Steps in Atheroma Lesion Formation [1–14]

Atheroma lesions have a spectrum of changes. Small localized raised foci in the young progress over years to form large areas of gruel and then go on to calcify and fibrose.

In the very young, the inner lining of arteries is smooth, elastic, and pliable. However, from the teens, or even earlier, onward, the inner surface develops small gray or white elevations, which are not very conspicuous on gross inspection. Some are so small that use of a magnifying glass is necessary for identification. When these lesions are processed, cut, stained, and examined with an ordinary light microscope, they show focal areas of damage to the inner wall of the artery. The damage consists of muscle cell damage together with edema in surrounding tissue. These particular lesions have been described by Daoud et al. [4] and Daria Haust [5], who mention early edematous and gelatinous lesions in children. This stage is followed by a cellular infiltrate of white blood cells, mainly macrophages and lymphocytes.

Small raised yellow elevations called fatty streaks appear. The *fatty streaks are seen microscopically* as a collection of fat-filled cells (foam cells, as they are called, on account of their foamy appearance). Using special stains, the different foam cells that make up the fatty streak lesion can be identified. As mentioned, one type of foam cell is a smooth muscle cell, a normal constituent of the artery. The other type is a macrophage or scavenger cell, derived from circulating white blood cells that infiltrate and take up fat in the artery wall.

As the lesion progresses, larger lesions are formed. Fatty streaks go on to form so-called fibronecrotic lipid plaques. The central necrotic core of these lesions consists of fatty granular gruel, accepted as inert fat and cholesterol, which is seen by electron microscopy as a conglomerate of small membranous vesicles and fatty droplets. As pointed out earlier, these vesicles are considered to be overlooked fatty *Chlamydia* germs.

The plaques progress to become either end-stage fibrosed calcified lesions containing fat, calcium, iron, and other constituents or hemorrhagic unstable lesions, which rupture into the lumen, causing clot formation and acute obstruction with dire consequences.

12.2. Aspects Requiring Reexamination

There are many unknowns about formation of these lesions that need explaining.

The beginning of the lesion has always been somewhat controversial. Various suggestions and postulates as to how the lesion starts have included endothelial damage, fat infiltration, infiltration of white cells, and proliferation of smooth muscle cells, among others. One could say that *ascertaining the initial change, the beginning, is a vital first step to unlocking the mystery of the lesion.*

Another aspect that needs attention concerns the reason for *arterial smooth muscle cells taking up fat and undergoing damage.* The normal artery contains muscle cells, which are contractile elements to keep the tone of the artery and accommodate variations in blood pressure. Muscle cells are not phagocytic, so why do they become infiltrated with fat and undergo damage? There is also a need to explain the reason for white blood cells, mainly *blood monocytes, attaching to and infiltrating into the artery, then changing into scavenger macrophages and taking up fat to become foam cells.*

A facet that has plagued all who have studied the lesion is the *mechanism involved in a fatty streak lesion progressing to form gruel-like fibronecrotic material.* How does a fatty cellular lesion become an acellular necrotic lesion?

Cholesterol is an aspect that has received great attention. The mechanism of deposition of cholesterol, and other fats, such as phospholipids, fatty acids, ceroid, a wax-like fatty substance, and nonmammalian fats, needs elucidation.

There is also the end-stage lesion: calcification, gradual fibrosis, and scar formation. Ulceration, hemorrhage, rupture, and clot formation are other features. These late changes appear to be nonspecific and to result from attempted healing, which is a feature of all chronic inflammatory and infective lesions.

12.3. Addressing the Problem of Atheroma Lesion Formation

To decipher this mysterious and evasive lesion and find answers to the unknown questions, it is necessary to examine the depths of the pathological features and find a novel method to look into all the unexplored dark nooks and crannies. Finding many of the lipid structures are actually *Chlamydia pneumoniae* germs introduces a new angle to the lesion. Instead of looking to explain how fat causes damage to the artery, one has to look if and how *Chlamydia* germs cause damage to the arteries.

Between one and two thousand arterial specimens containing all stages of atheroma lesions were received for examination each year. The large number of specimens allowed an in depth study to determine how *Chlamydia* germs primarily infect arteries and go through various steps, to colonize and form necrotic atheroma gruel.

For light microscopy, in addition to the usual stains such as hematoxylin and eosin, Masson trichrome stain, and Giemsa, selected cases were also stained with immunoperoxidase for smooth muscle actin, macrophage CD68, and *Chlamydia* monoclonal antibody. For electron microscopy, thin slivers of tissue were cut with a special machine, then placed on special copper grids, stained, and then examined.

New findings require some type of documentation or proof. Photographs showing all the various aspects of the lesion had to be produced. Photographs are irrefutable visual evidence of what happens and how damage and destruction occur. It was necessary to prove beyond reasonable doubt the exact cause of destruction to arteries before a formal charge of malicious damage to property, let alone the capital charge of murder and genocide of the human race, could be leveled and submitted for consideration and judgment.

Is it really possible that a little germ is responsible for all the upheaval and pathological changes that occur in formation of the atheroma lesion?

Although a lengthy search looking down an electron microscope may seem a boring and mundane type of task, the fact of the matter is, that when one is looking and discovering new things, even in the minute world, there is some excitement and anticipation, probably no less intense than in discovering new uncharted things in the macro-world.

References

1. Aldons JL. Atheroscleosis. Nature (Lond) 2000;407:233–241.
2. Benditt EP, Schwartz SM. Blood vessels. In: Rubin E, Farber JL (eds) Pathology. Philadelphia: Lippincott, 1989:459–467.
3. Davies MJ, Woolf N. Atherosclerosis: what is it and why does it occur. Br Heart J 1993;69(suppl):S3–S11.
4. Daoud AJ, Jarmolych A, Zumbo R, et al. Pre-atheroma phase of coronary atherosclerosis in man. Exp Mol Pathol 1964;3:475–484.
5. Haust D. The morphogenesis and fate of potential and early atherosclerotic lesions in man. Hum Pathol 1971;1(2):1–29.
6. Libby P, Ridker PM, Maseri A. Inflammation and atherosclerosis. Circulation 2002;105:1135–1143.
7. Libby P, Hansson GK. Involvement of the immune system in human atherogenesis: Current knowledge and unanswered questions. Lab Invest 1991;64(1):5–15.
8. Ross R. Atherosclerosis. In: McGee JO, Isaacson PG, Wright NA (eds) Oxford textbook of pathology. New York: Oxford University Press 1992;2A:798–811.
9. Gaudio E, Carpino G, Grassi M, Musca A. Morphological aspects of atherosclerotic lesion: past and present. Clin Ter 2006;157(2):135–142.
10. Stary HC, Blankenhorn DH, Chandler B, et al. A definition of intima of human arteries and of its atherosclerosis-prone regions. Circulation 1992;85(1):391–405.

11. Stary HC, Chandler AB, Glacov S, et al. A definition of initial fatty streak, and intermediate lesions of atherosclerosis. A report from the committee on vascular lesions of the council on atherosclerosis, American Heart Association. Arterioscler Thromb 1994;14:840–856.
12. Stary HC, Chandler AB, Dismore RE, et al. A definition of advanced types of atherosclerotic lesions and histological classification of atherosclerosis. A report from the Committee on Vascular Lesions of the Council of Atherosclerosis, American Heart Association. Circulation 1995;92:1355–1374.
13. Mc Gill HC Jr. Persistent problems in the pathogenesis of atherosclerosis. Arteriosclerosis 1984;4:443–451.
14. Geer JC, McGill HC Jr, Robertson WB, et al. Histological characteristics of coronary artery fatty streaks. Lab Invest 1968;18(5):105–110.

13 New Findings Concerning the Initial Lesion

Chlamydia germs damage arteries

Let us press on to the findings of the study. Reexamination of the pathological features, with due consideration for the presence of *Chlamydia* organisms, opened up new insights into the lesion.

13.1. Initial Lesion

Possibly the most important aspect in solving the many mysteries of lesion formation lies in defining the initial damage, the beginning, the very first microscopic pathological change that occurs. The beginning is the key to opening the door to the progressive steps of lesion formation.

Atheroma lesions begin in the inner layer of the artery, or intima, as it is called. The contents of this layer are fairly simple, consisting of only three components: loose connective tissue and smooth muscle cells covered by a single layer of flat endothelial cells on the lumen side.

It seems easy enough to look at each of these components and determine where, what, and how the damage commences. But this has proved to be not so easy. In fact, determination of the locality and constitution of the initial lesion has been elusive and clouded in controversy.

Nonpathological studies view the lesion as beginning with primary damage to the lining endothelial cells, that is, damage to the barrier separating the inner artery from the blood. After all, how else to explain the phenomenon of lipid and cellular infiltrate from the blood, into the artery, other than by some defect in this barrier [1–4] [see also references in Chapter 12]. Although there is obviously some mechanism that allows infiltration of cells into the artery, *pathological studies accept that the endothelium is intact and there is no physical damage to this layer seen by microscopy or electron microscopy* [see Chapter 3: references 15, 16, 40].

13.2. Primary Muscle Damage [5–12]

So, if the endothelium is intact and shows no visible damage, where then does the primary damage to the artery occur? Other than endothelium, only underlying smooth muscle cells and connective tissue are present. We therefore have to turn our attention to these components.

13.2.1. Light Microscopy

Examination of very small early lesions, with a light microscope, shows that *primary damage takes place in the muscle cell component of the intima.* The cells become vacuolated, accumulate lipid, swell, fragment, and necrose. The inner layer of the artery takes on a moth-eaten appearance because of the damage and eventual loss of muscle cells (Figures 13.1–13.4).

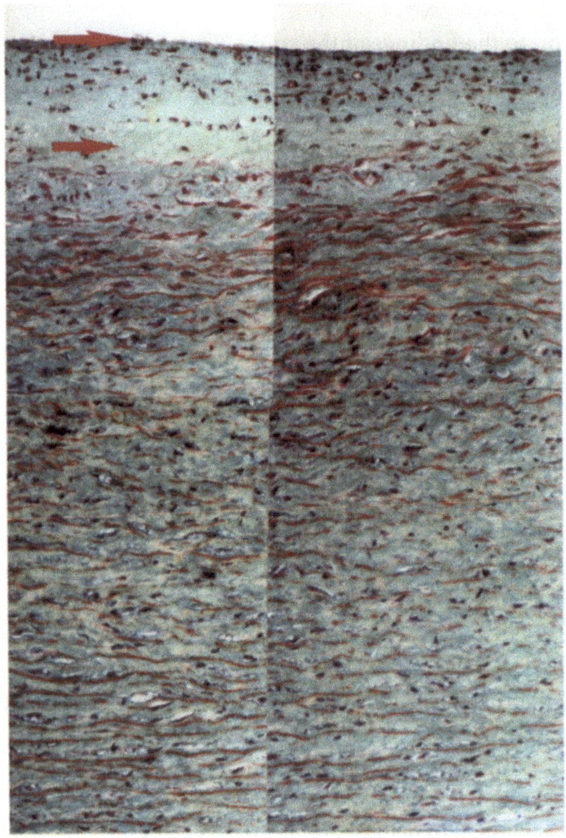

Figure 13.1. Micrograph of artery wall. Montage of section of aorta shows the artery wall consists mainly of media layer (muscle cells and elastic tissue) and inner layer or intima in upper micrograph (demarcated by *arrows*). Masson stain.

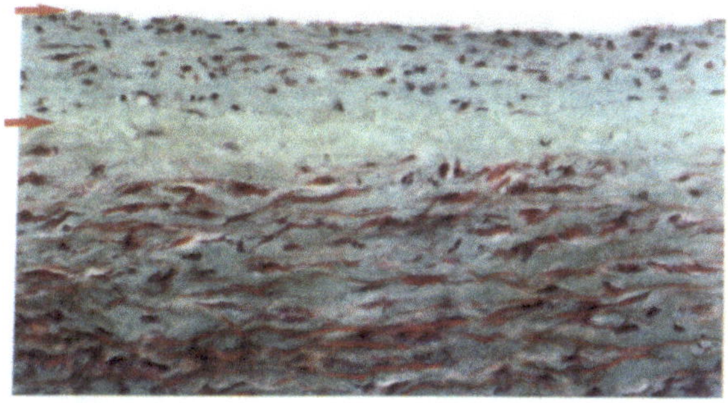

Figure 13.2. Micrograph of normal inner layer (intima of artery). Micrograph of section of normal arterial intima, consisting of connective tissue and muscle cells (area demarcated by *arrows*). ×100.

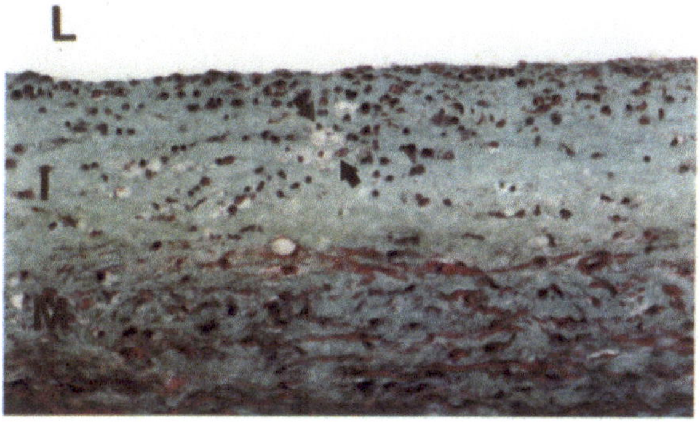

Figure 13.3. Early damage to inner layer (intima). Micrograph of section of artery lumen (*L*). *I*, intima; *M*, media. Early damage of intimal muscle cells is seen as small lucent foci in the intima layer (*arrows*). ×100.

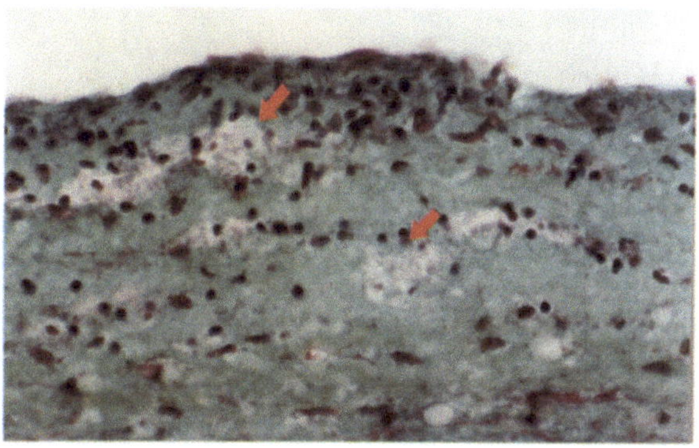

Figure 13.4. Damaged muscle cells in inner layer in greater detail. Enlargement of section of intima shows damaged muscle cells, which appear as clear areas (*arrows*). ×400.

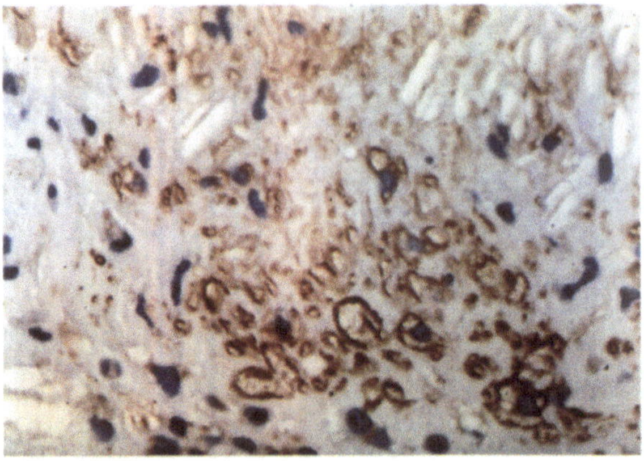

Figure 13.5. Immunoperoxidase staining of damaged muscle cells. Special stain (immunoperoxidase smooth muscle actin) shows damaged muscle cells in intima. (Smooth muscle components stain *brown*.)

It is not difficult to identify damage occurring in intimal muscle cells, as the cells stain positive with specific immunocytochemical stain for smooth muscle actin (Figure 13.5).

The damaged muscle cells also contain fine sand-like granules in the cytoplasm, which are confirmed to be *Chlamydia* germs by use of a special immunocytochemical stain (Figures 13.6, 13.7).

Infection and destruction of single muscle cells are described, but with progression more and more muscle cells become destroyed, producing larger areas of intimal damage and muscle loss (Figure 13.8).

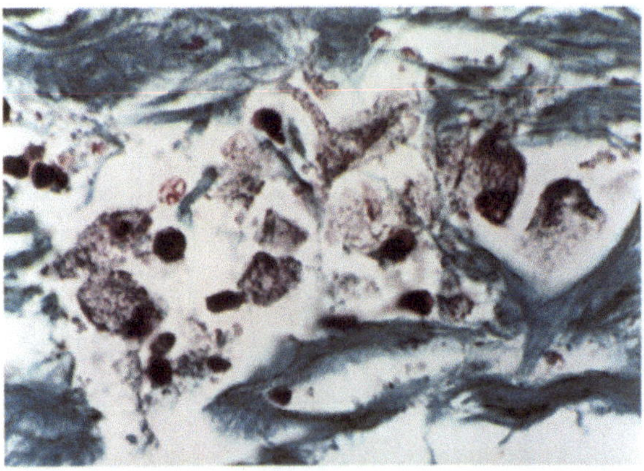

Figure 13.6. Damaged muscle cells contain granular material. A little more detail of the damaged muscle cells showing fine sand-like granular material in cell cytoplasm. ×400.

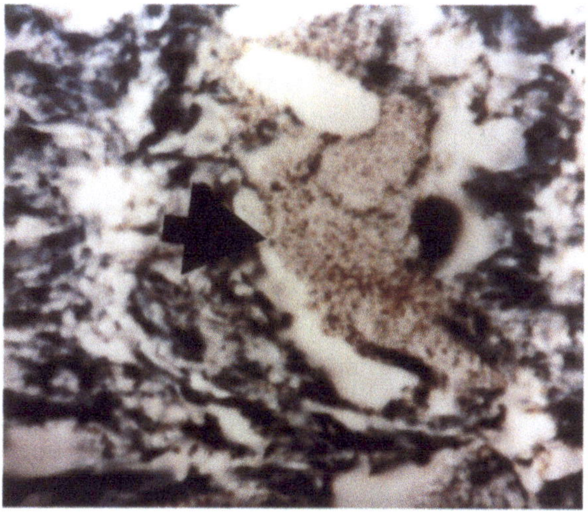

Figure 13.7. Muscle cells contain fine sand-like *Chlamydia* inclusions. Micrograph of damaged muscle cell shows fine sand-like *Chlamydia* material in the cytoplasm (*arrow*). ×1000.

13.2.2. Electron Microscopy

Looking at the muscle damage under the electron microscope shows the process in greater detail.

Elongated smooth muscle cells are identified by the presence of myofibrils, which are string-like contractile elements found in the cytoplasm of smooth muscle cells. Other identifying features of muscle cells such as basement membrane material and dense bodies are sometimes also noted.

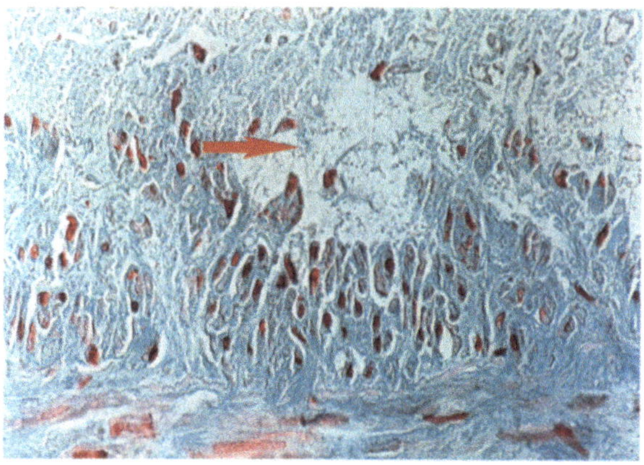

Figure 13.8. Larger focal area of muscle damage of intima. Micrograph shows extension of muscle damage. Lucent area resulting from muscle loss (*arrow*). Note loss of muscle cells. This lesion is similar to the early edematous lesion described by Daoud et al. [see Chapter 12: reference 4].

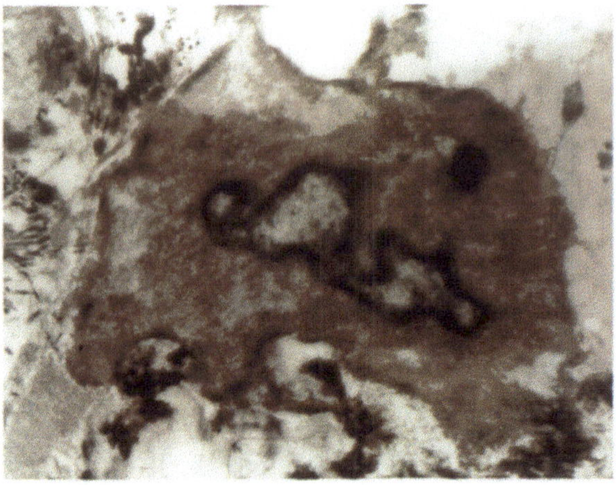

Figure 13.9. Electron micrograph shows normal intimal muscle cell.

Muscle cells contain vacuoles with Chlamydia *germs.*

Germs and vacuoles grow and increase in size, destroying and displacing much of the cytoplasm and myofibrils.

The cell is eventually unable to contain the sheer bulk and expansive growth of the organisms and vacuoles. *Highly vacuolated infected and damaged muscle cells start fragmenting and disintegrating, resulting in complete destruction of the cell.*

The contents are released and *germs, fat, and muscle fragments are dispersed into the surrounding extracellular tissue* (Figures 13.9–13.17).

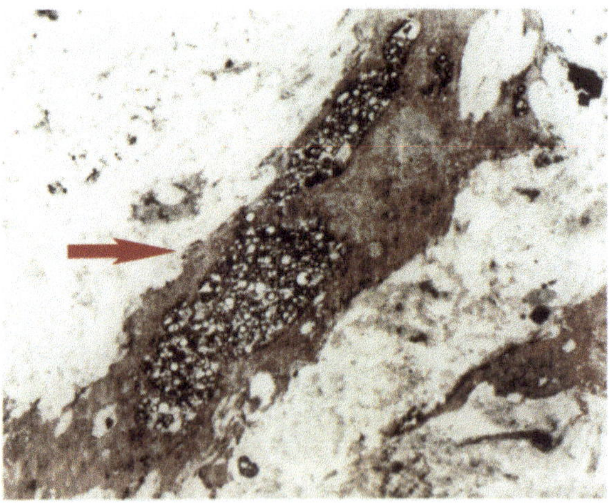

Figure 13.10. Electron micrograph shows infected muscle cell (*arrow*) containing *Chlamydia* (small dark structures in cytoplasm).

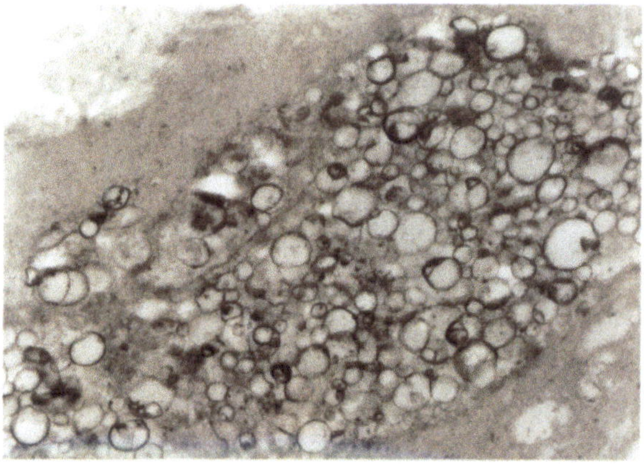

Figure 13.11. Infected muscle cell in greater detail. Electron micrograph shows greater magnification and more detail of infected muscle cell. Multiple *Chlamydia* organisms replace the muscle cell cytoplasm.

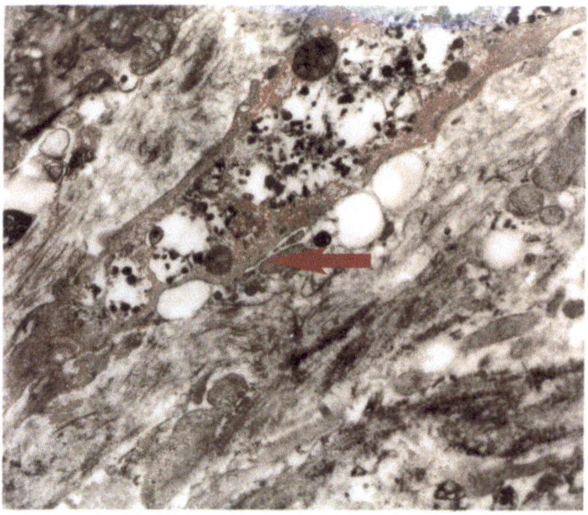

Figure 13.12. Damaged muscle cell. Electron micrograph shows infected and damaged smooth muscle cell (*arrow*). Cell has been destroyed by vacuoles and germs.

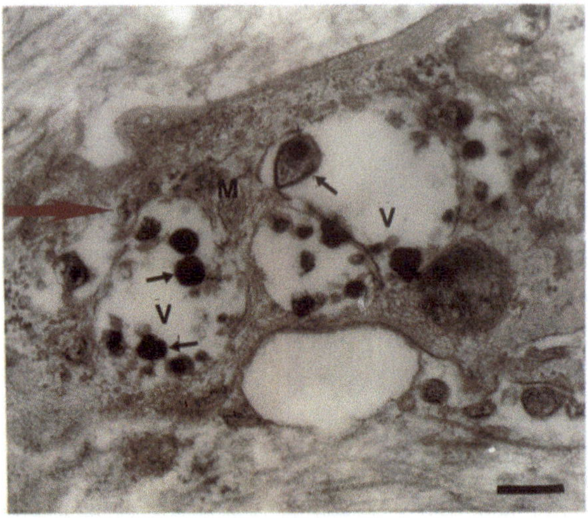

Figure 13.13. Damaged muscle cell in greater detail. Electron micrograph with greater enlargement shows muscle cell in more detail (*red arrow*). Note string-like myofibrils in cytoplasm (*M*) and *Chlamydia* organisms (*black arrows*) in vacuoles (*V*). The electron micrograph shows how germs grow in vacuoles and replace and destroy much of the cytoplasm and myofibrils. (Electron micrograph reprinted from Shor A, Phillips I, Ong G, et al. [see Chapter 10: reference 4], with permission from the *Journal of Clinical Pathology*, Blackwell Publishers.)

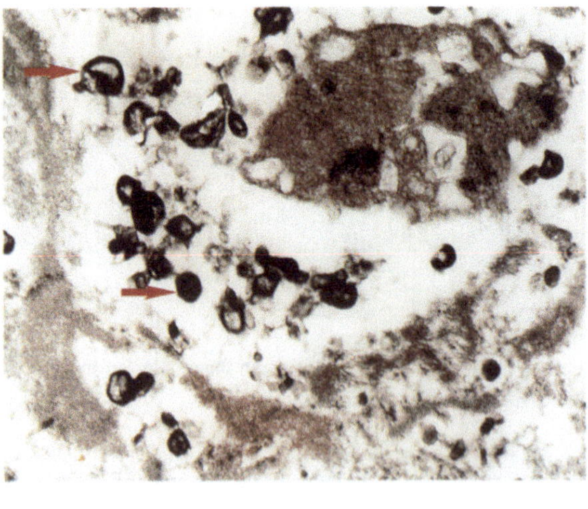

Figure 13.14. Fragmenting muscle cell. Electron micrograph shows destruction of muscle cell with rupture and release of dark irregular *Chlamydia* structures into the extracellular space (*arrows*).

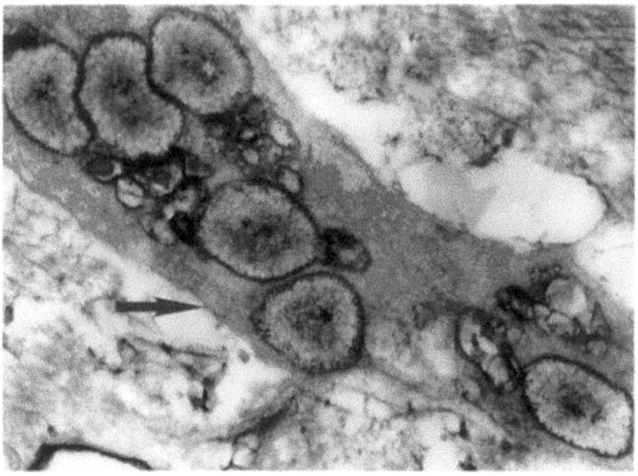

Figure 13.15. Another infected muscle cell. Muscle cell (*arrow*) containing larger reticulate bodies, with smaller elementary bodies. (From Shor et al. [6], with permission from the *Cardiovascular Journal of South Africa*.)

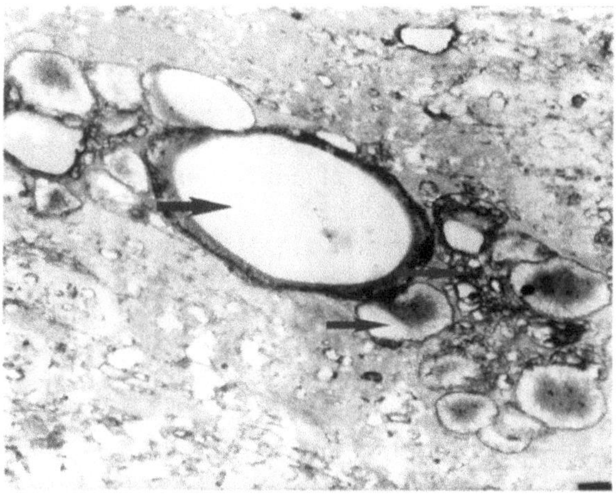

Figure 13.16. Fragmenting muscle cell. Electron micrograph of fragmenting muscle cell containing a large clear vacuole, intermediate-sized reticulate bodies with central dense core, and multiple small elementary bodies (*arrows*).

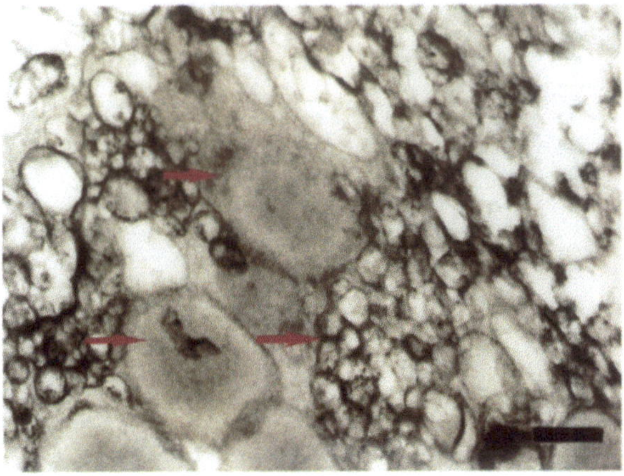

Figure 13.17. Dispersion of germs. Electron micrograph shows dispersion of organisms after rupture of the cell. Gruel contains similar larger reticulate bodies, and a collection of smaller elementary bodies (*arrows*). The last three electron micrographs illustrate infection, damage, fragmentation, and dissemination of germs (see previous electron micrographs, Figures 13.15 and 13.14).

13.3. *Chlamydia* Cause Muscle Cell Damage

The larger areas of damage and loss of muscle cells are similar to the early focal edematous intimal lesions, described in the 1960s and 1970s by Daoud et al. and Haust [see Chapter 12: references 4, 5]. At the time, the lesion was described as a lucent or edematous area of the intima, with an unknown cause. The lesion did not receive much prominence, being overshadowed by fat deposition in the artery.

A few previous studies that have looked at the phenomenon of muscle damage postulate that it may be fat that somehow damages the muscle cells. Another suggestion is that damage may be caused by hemodynamic factors with mechanical disruption of cells, related to increased blood pressure [13].

Finding *Chlamydia* germs in muscle cells adds a new dimension to the mechanism and cause of muscle damage. The process is one of infection, damage, disintegration of muscle cells, and dispersion of organisms.

Chlamydia as a group are pathogenic germs that have a propensity to infect and damage cells. As obligate intracellular organisms, they vegetate and grow in intracytoplasmic vacuoles. Growth and enlargement of vacuoles result in damage to cytoplasm with rupture of the cell and dispersion of organisms [see Chapter 6: reference 1].

Arterial muscle damage is therefore seen as physical damage, with the cell being unable to contain the continued growth of *Chlamydia* germs, and expansion of vacuoles in which they live.

References

1. Gresham GA. Early events in atherogenesis. Lancet 1975;1(7907):614–615.
2. Luscher TF, Noll G. The pathogenesis of cardiovascular disease: role of the endothelium as a target and mediator. Atherosclerosis 1995;118:S81–S90.
3. Zither AM. Endothelium vasodilator dysfunction: pathogenic link to myocardial ischaemia or epiphenomenon. Lancet 1996;348:S10–S12.
4. Noll G, Luscher TE. Influence of lipoproteins on endothelial function. Thromb Res 1994;74:S45–S54.
5. Shor A. Early intimal smooth muscle cell necrosis in atherosclerosis. Presented at the 34th Annual Congress of the South African Society of Pathology, 3–6 July, !994.
6. Shor A, Phillips JI. Histological and ultra structural findings suggesting an initiating role for *Chlamydia pneumoniae* in the pathogenesis of atherosclerosis. Cardiovasc J S Afr 2000;11(1):16–23.
7. Shor A. Method of arterial infection by *Chlamydia pneumoniae.* (Letter.) Circulation 2001;104(13):E75.
8. Shor A. The pathology of *Chlamydia pneumoniae* in humans and animal models. Trends Microbiol 2000;8(12):541.
9. Shor A. A pathologist's view of organisms and human atherosclerosis. J Infect Dis 2001;183(9):1428–1429.
10. Shor A, Phillips I. *Chlamydia pneumoniae* and atherosclerosis. JAMA 1999; 282(21):2071–2073.
11. Shor A, Walker ARP, Ballard R, et al. Changing concepts of coronary artery disease. Part 1. Round -table discussion on factors playing a role in atherosclerosis. Cardiovasc J S Afr 2000;11(1):32–40.
12. Shor A, Walker ARP, Ballard R, et al. Changing concepts of coronary artery disease. Part 2. Round -table discussion. Cardiovasc J S Afr 2000;11(3):161–168.
13. Stehbens WE. The elusive factor in atherosclerosis. Med Hypotheses 1997; 48(6):503–509.

14
Fatty Streak Lesion

Cells versus germ

14.1. Macrophage Infiltration

If there was no resistance, attack by germs would continue unabated until complete destruction of the artery occurred. Luckily, the body has some defense mechanisms to counteract foreign invaders. Different cellular, inflammatory, and immunological mechanisms come into play in reaction to invasion and damage by germs.

So let us look into the next stage of the lesion, namely, the cellular response, which aggregates at the site of infection and helps in the body's defense against the virulent germs.

14.2. Macrophages Phagocytose Fat, Germs, and Muscle

Use of cell-specific monoclonal antibodies has permitted an accurate delineation of the composition of each of the different cell types that help with defense. It has been shown that there is increased adherence of blood monocytes in clusters onto the endothelial lining. Chemotactic factors induce the monocytes to penetrate actively between the endothelial cells and migrate to the subendothelial space. Many of the monocytes become active as macrophages and, in their role as scavenger cells, attempt to remove deleterious material, germs, and fat [1–5].

14.2.1. Light Microscopy

Monocytes attach to the endothelium, infiltrate into the intima, and go on to form macrophages, which enlarge, take up fat, and form a mass of fat-laden foam cells. The cellular reaction occurs in relation to damaged intimal muscle cells (Figures 14.1–14.3).

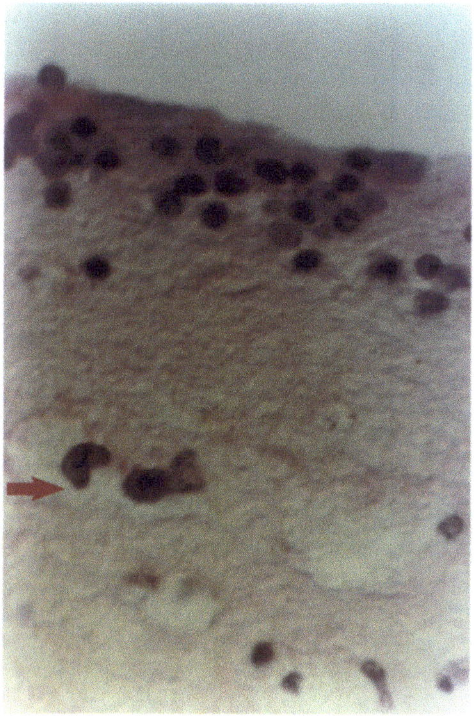

Figure 14.1. Blood monocytes infiltrating artery. Micrograph shows cluster of blood monocytes infiltrating into the subendothelial space of an artery. Note underlying vacuolated muscle cell (*arrow*). ×400.

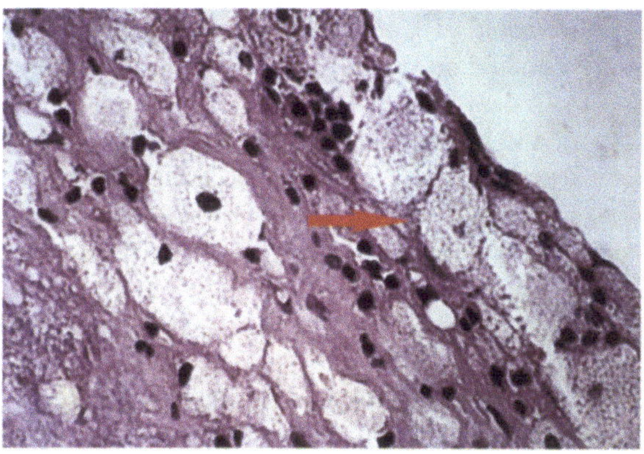

Figure 14.2. Monocytes change to macrophage/foam cells. Micrograph shows later stage in which monocytes have enlarged, changed to form macrophage/foam cells, and migrated deeper into the intima. Cells contain fat and granular material (*arrow*). ×400.

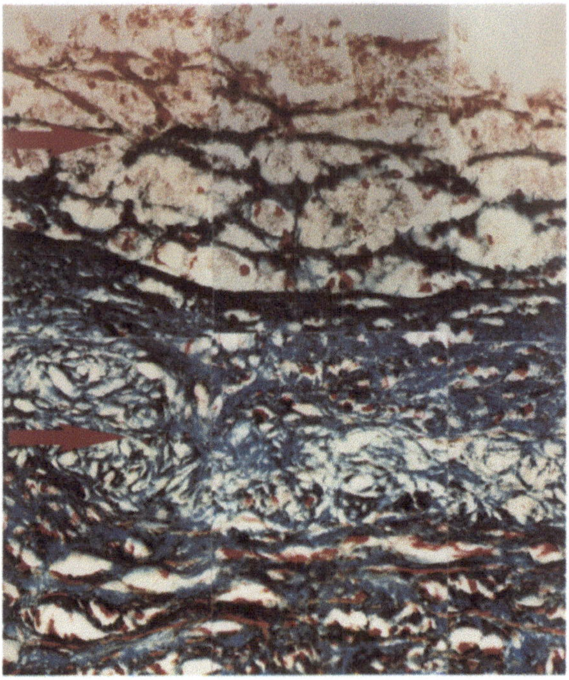

FIGURE 14.3. Micrograph shows foam cells in relation to damaged muscle cells. Micrograph of fatty streak lesion shows clear foam cells (*arrows*) with underlying area of damaged muscle cells (*arrow*).

The foam cells are noted to contain not only *fat*, but *also fine granular material, shown to be* Chlamydia *organisms* using special immunocytochemical stains [6].

In addition to fat and germs, glycogen granules start appearing in the cytoplasm. *Glycogen* deposition is a feature of *Chlamydia trachomatis*-infected cells, but this has not been described in *Chlamydia pneumoniae*-infected cells. So here is a point of interest concerning the *Chlamydia* germ of atheroma (Figure 14.4).

Another undescribed feature of the macrophage/foam cell infiltrate is that some of these cells fuse together and form *multinucleate giant cells, which wrap around and try to engulf* Chlamydia-*infected muscle cells* (Figure 14.5).

14.2.2. Electron Microscopy

Macrophage cells are found in areas of muscle damage where they are seen to engulf and contain not only fat, but also muscle fragments and *Chlamydia* germs (Figures 14.6–14.9).

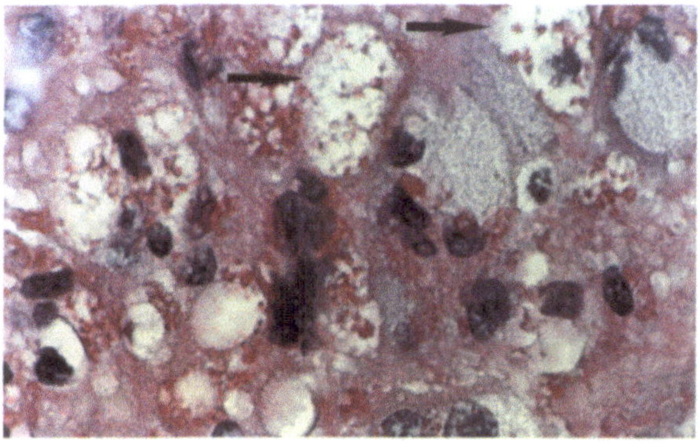

Figure 14.4. Cellular reaction to damage. Micrograph shows clear foam cells containing fat and glycogen (*red-stained* material; *arrows*) adjacent to granular infected muscle cells (cells with gray fine sand-like inclusion bodies). Periodic acid–Schiff (PAS) stain. ×400.

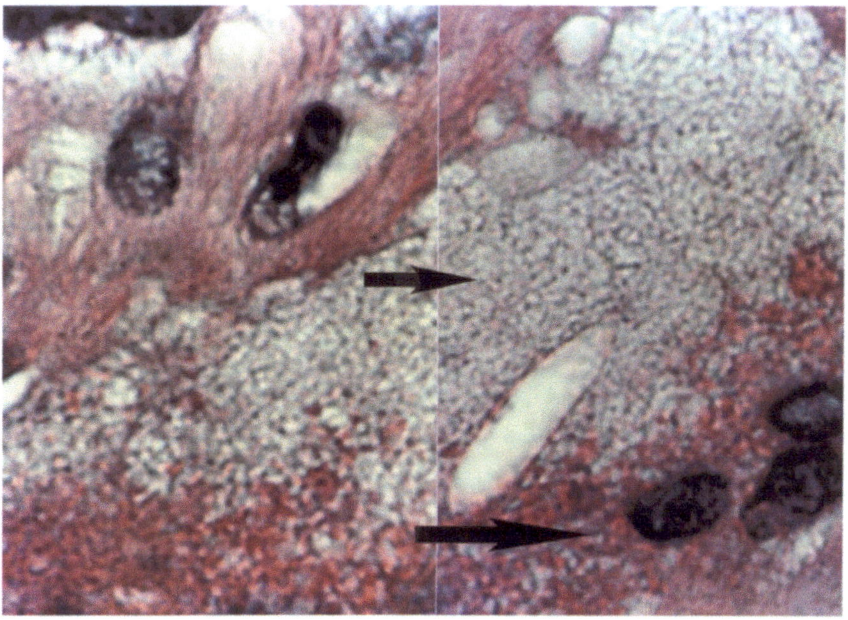

Figure 14.5. Micrograph showing macrophages attack infected muscle cell and germs. Montage micrograph shows infected muscle cell, containing gray sand-like *Chlamydia* inclusions (*arrow*), being enveloped by a multinucleate macrophage giant cell containing multiple nuclei and red-staining glycogen droplets (*arrow*). The multinucleate cell is attacking the *Chlamydia*-infected cell, trying to engulf and destroy the hostile organisms. This picture conveys the process of infected muscle cells being attacked by macrophage/giant cells. PAS stain. ×1000.

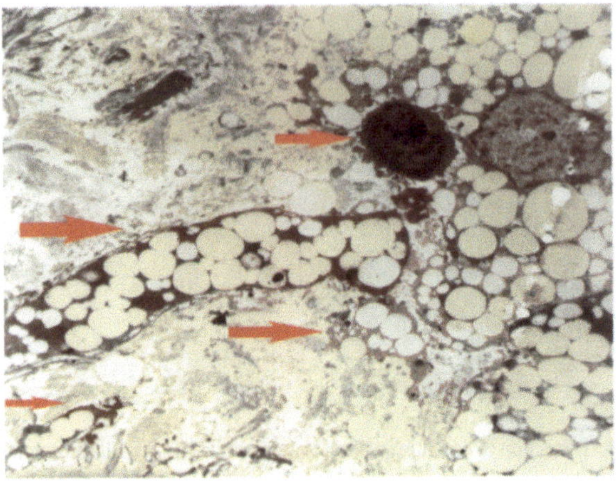

Figure 14.6. Electron micrograph. Foam cells engulfing muscle fragment. Transmission electron micrograph shows foam cell engulfing elongated muscle cell fragments and nucleus (*arrows*).

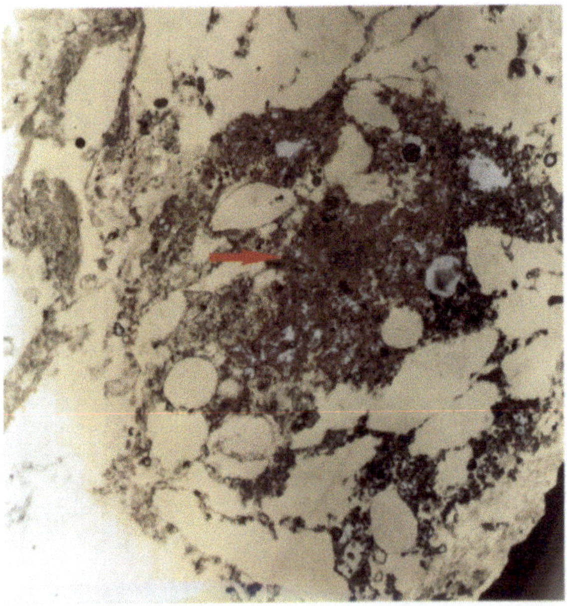

Figure 14.7. Electron micrograph. Foam cells contain muscle fragments. Transmission electron micrograph shows foam cell containing degenerate muscle fragment (*arrow*).

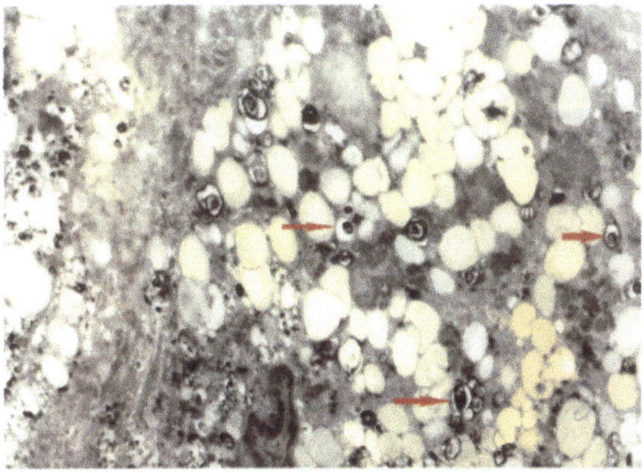

Figure 14.8. Electron micrograph. Foam cells also contain *Chlamydia* organisms. Transmission electron micrograph shows foam cell containing multiple small dense *Chlamydia* organisms (*arrows*).

14.3. Macrophage Reaction Resulting from Germs and Muscle Damage

The exact cause of the macrophage infiltrate has been a source of some debate. Blood monocytes originate in bone marrow and lymphoid tissue and change to become phagocytic macrophages, to form part of the normal cellular

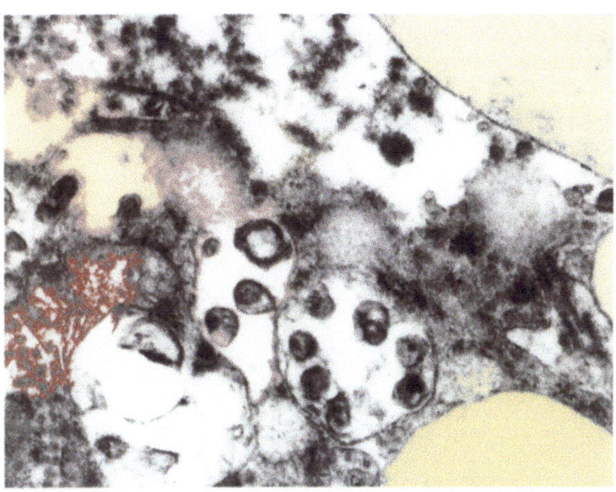

Figure 14.9. Electron micrograph of *Chlamydia* in foam cells. Transmission electron micrograph. Higher magnification shows details of pear-shaped *Chlamydia* germs in foam cell. (From Kuo C-C, Shor A, Campbell LA, et al. [see Chapter 8: reference 3], with permission from the *Journal of Infectious Diseases*.)

reaction, which occurs in response to foreign material or invaders that enter the artery.

As the macrophages are seen to pick up germs, lipid, and damaged muscle fragments, they are *viewed as a secondary response to mop up the germs, lipid, and damaged muscle cells.*

The cell reaction is similar to that which occurs in other *Chlamydia* infections, where a prominent macrophage reaction forms part of the lesion.

References

1. Gowen AM, Tsukada T, Ross R. Immunocytochemical analysis of the cellular composition of human atherosclerotic lesions. Am J Pathol 1986;125:191–207.
2. Roessner A, Herrera A, Honing HJ, et al. Identification of macrophages and smooth muscle cells with monoclonal antibodies in the human atherosclerotic plaque. Virchows Arch A Pathol Anat Histopathol 1987;412(2):169–174.
3. Li AC, Glass CK. The macrophage foam cell as target for therapeutic intervention. Nat Med 2002;8:S1235–S1241.
4. Gerrity RG. The role of the monocyte in atherogenesis. Am J Pathol 1981;103: 191–200.
5. Airenne S, Surcel HM, Lakarpa H, et al. *Chlamydia pneumoniae* infection in human monocytes. Infect Immun 1999;67(3):1445–1449.
6. Kuo C-C, Gowan AM, Benditt ER. Detection of *Chlamydia pneumoniae* in aortic lesions by immunocytochemical stain. Arterioscler Thromb 1993;13:1501–1504.

15
Formation of Fibronecrotic Plaque

Strange new findings

The next stage occurs when the fatty streak lesion progresses to form a mass of necrotic atheroma gruel, the so-called fibronecrotic plaque.

Studies have suggested that foam cells lead to formation of much of the gruel material, but there has been some difficulty in explaining how large fat droplets, which make up most of the fat in foam cells, change to become multiple small membranous structures in atheroma gruel [1] (Figures 15.1, 15.2).

There are other questions, related to gruel formation, such as the origin of ceroid bodies and cholesterol crystals, which occur in increasing quantities as the lesion progresses.

The late sequelae of the gruel, such as fibrosis, calcification, hemorrhage, and rupture, also require explanation.

15.11 Formation of Atheroma Gruel

15.1.1. Light Microscopy

Light microscopy shows that foam cells of the fatty streak lesion contain fine sand-like granular material. The cells appear to enlarge, rupture, and release the granular contents into the interstitium to form atheroma gruel (Figures 15.3–15.6).

15.1.2. Electron Microscopy

Multiple fatty structures in foam cells were examined in some detail to determine the process by which they form small membranous structures.

Scrutiny showed that some large fat structures in the foam cells are actually vacuoles in which organisms grow and proliferate. It was noted that some of the vacuoles develop small dense structures in the outer membrane, which go

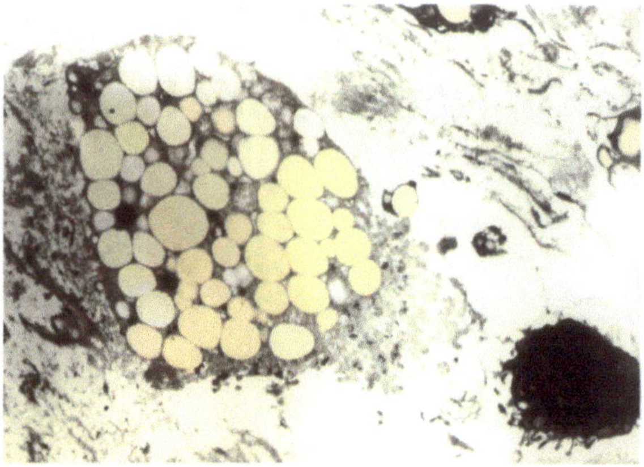

Figure 15.1. Electron micrograph. Foam cells contain large fat droplets. Transmission electron micrograph shows fragmenting foam cell containing large fat droplets. Note separating nucleus.

on to sporulate, bud, and produce multiple round, pear-shaped, and other forms of *Chlamydia* elementary bodies.

The process is similar to the described *Chlamydia* intracellular vegetative cycle that takes place entirely within a membrane-limited inclusion vacuole, and is considered analogous to bacterial sporulation.

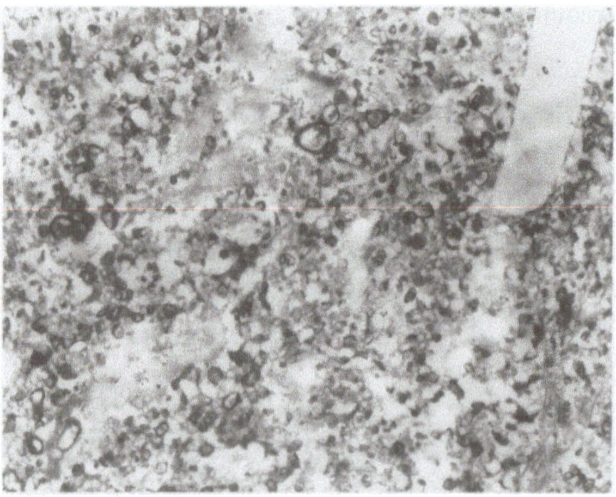

Figure 15.2. Electron micrograph. Small fatty membranous structures in atheroma gruel. Transmission electron micrograph of small membranous structures of atheroma gruel. The question is: How do large fat structures in foam cell (see previous electron micrograph) form a conglomerate of small membranous structures?

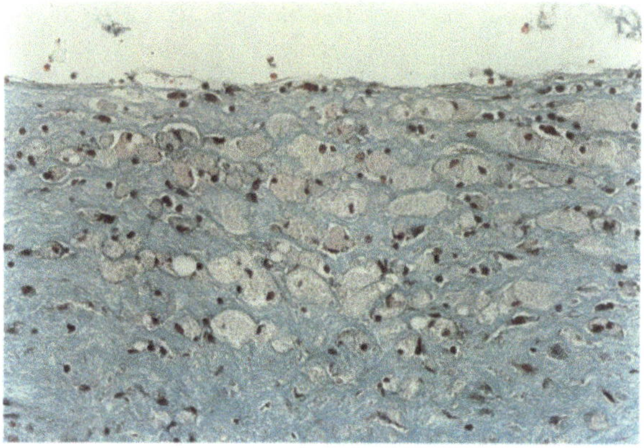

Figure 15.3. Micrograph. Foam cells in artery. Micrograph of fatty streak lesion shows collection of foam cells in intima. Cells contain fine sand-like granules in cytoplasm. Masson stain. ×100.

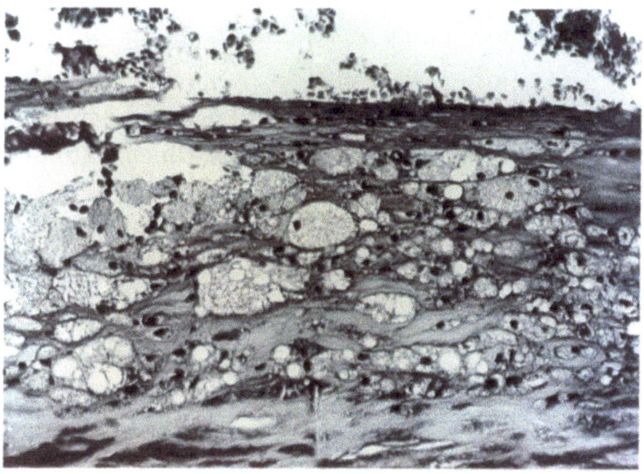

Figure 15.4. Fragmenting foam cells. Micrograph shows foam cells of various sizes; some are fragmenting. ×100.

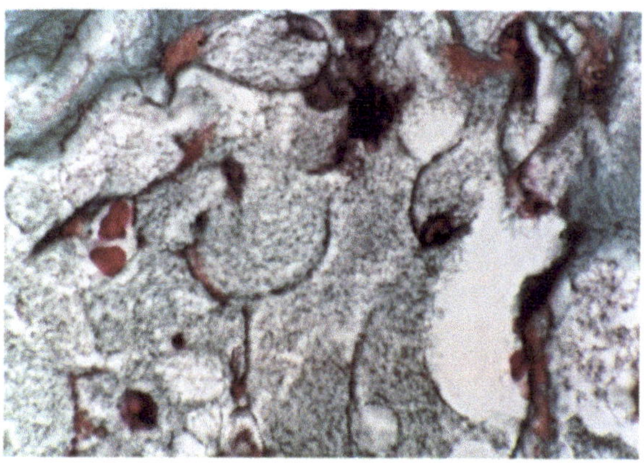

Figure 15.5. Fragmenting foam cells, releasing granules. Micrograph shows fragmented foam cells with release of fine sand-like granular contents. Masson stain. ×800.

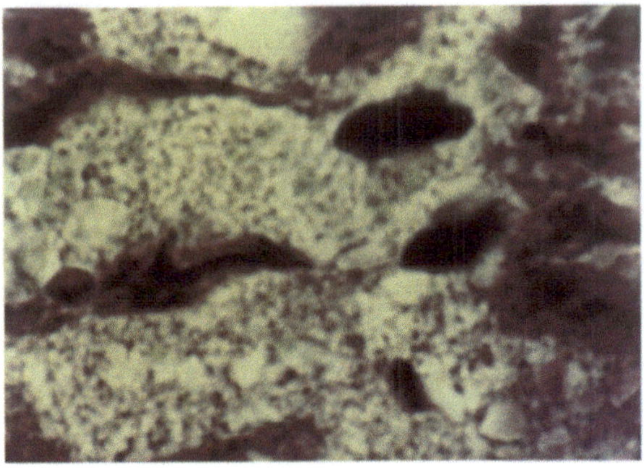

Figure 15.6. Released granules that make up atheroma gruel. Micrograph shows released granules. Giemsa stain. ×1000.

The cell ultimately ruptures with resultant release and dispersion of its contents, lipid, *Chlamydia* organisms, and vacuoles, which go to form much of the atheroma gruel (Figures 15.7–15.14).

The findings suggest *atheroma gruel is formed by a process of intracellular proliferation of* Chlamydia *germs, followed by fragmentation and rupture of the cells with dispersion and deposition of the germs.*

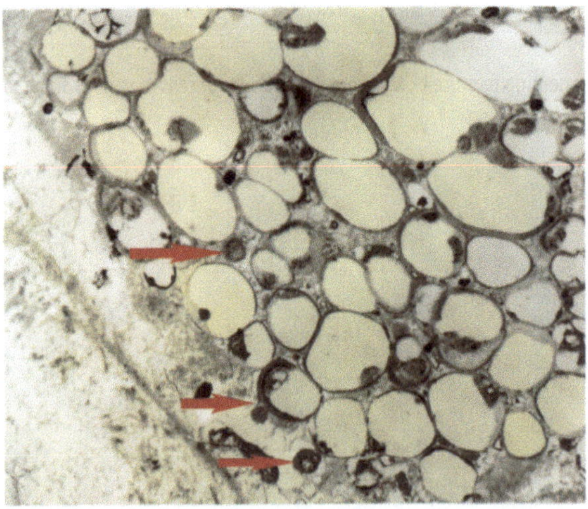

Figure 15.7. Vacuoles in foam cells starting to bud. Electron micrograph of a foam cell shows vacuoles forming electron-dense material (*arrows*).

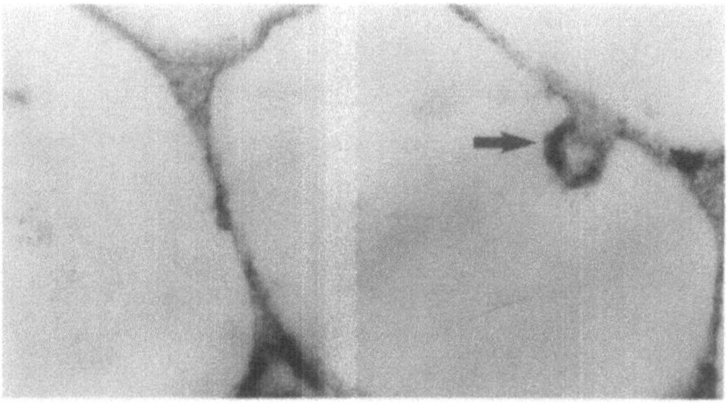

Figure 15.8. Vacuoles starting to form organisms. Transmission electron micrograph shows budding structure developing in vacuolar membrane (*arrow*).

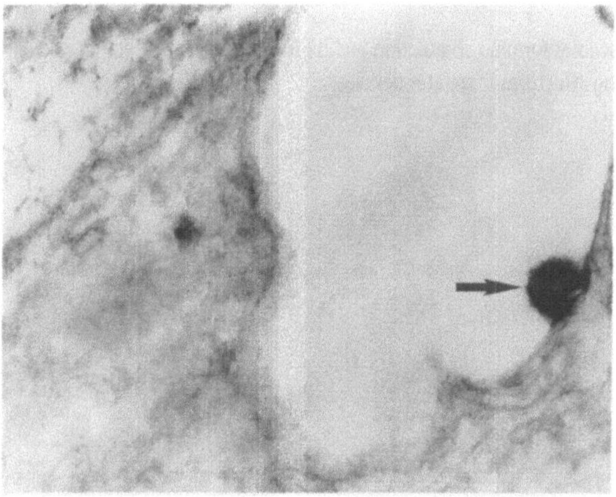

Figure 15.9. Vacuoles starting to form organisms. Transmission electron micrograph shows budding dense structure in vacuole membrane (*arrow*).

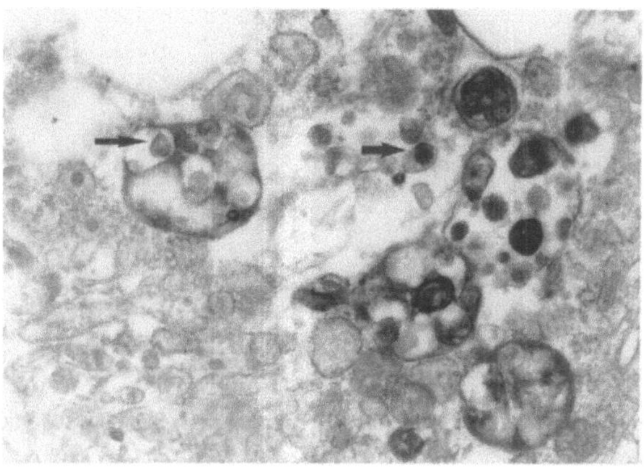

Figure 15.10. Sporulating structures in vacuole. Transmission electron micrograph shows formation of sporulating structures and budding pear-shaped structures in vacuole (*arrows*).

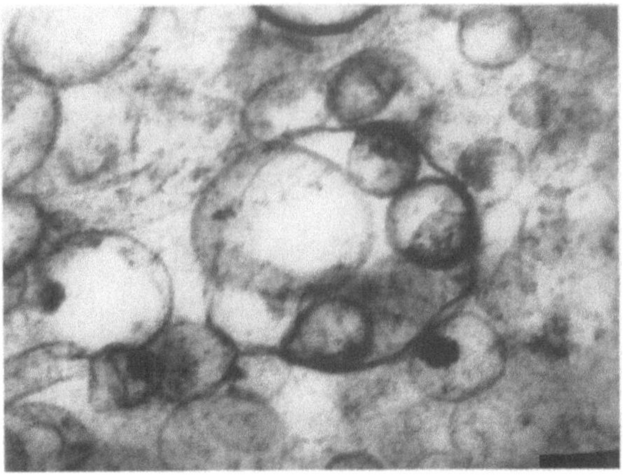

Figure 15.11. Vacuoles forming sporulating and budding organisms. Electron micrograph shows sporulating and budding structures in greater detail.

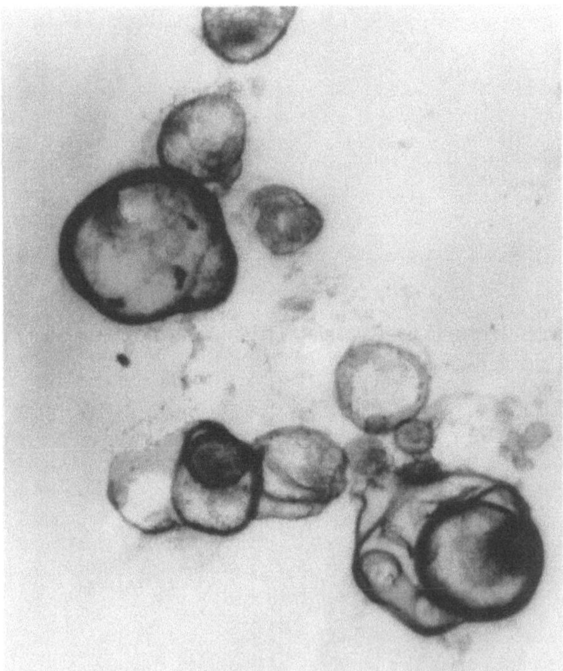

Figure 15.12. Formation of dividing structures. Electron micrograph shows collection of dividing and budding structures.

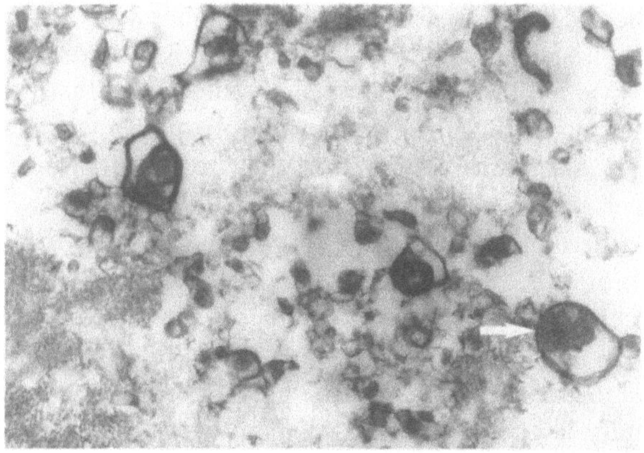

Figure 15.13. Gruel containing budding *Chlamydia* structures. Transmission electron micrograph shows membranous structures of atheroma gruel with budding structure (*arrow*). (Reprinted from Shor A, Kuo C-C, Patton DL [see Chapter 8: reference 1], with permission from the *South African Medical Journal*.)

15.2. Ceroid or Blighted *Chlamydia* Vacuoles?

Ceroid is a lipoprotein. Its basic components are unsaturated fatty acid esters that have undergone oxidation and polymerization. These structures, which occur in increasing amounts as the lesion progresses, have not received much prominence, yet they are inherent components of the gruel and deserve some explanation for their presence [2,3].

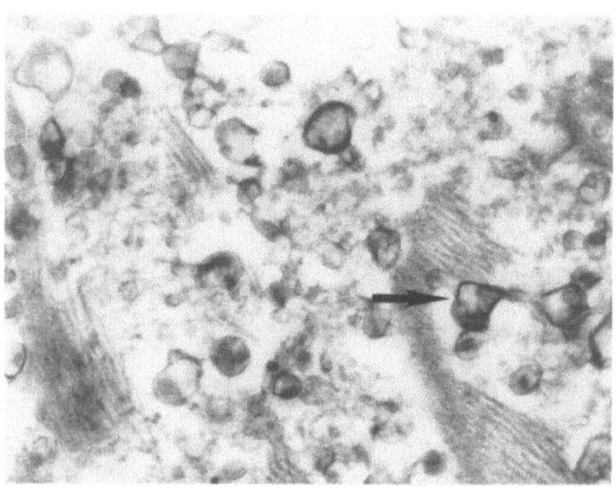

Figure 15.14. Gruel containing dividing *Chlamydia* structures. Electron micrograph of atheroma gruel shows dividing structures (*arrow*).

Microscopically, they appear as wavy membranous deep red structures when atheroma gruel is stained with Masson trichrome. By electron microscopy they are seen as wavy, multilamellar, laminated structures. What is strange about ceroid in atheroma is that the electron microscopic appearance of irregular, laminated wavy structures is different from the appearance of conventional ceroid found elsewhere in the body.

Ceroid in atheroma appears to be formed in the following manner. With disintegration of cells, there is dispersion of fat, germs, and also the vacuoles in which the germs live. The released vacuoles in the extracellular tissue appear to go on to grow and form large wavy membranous multilamellar ceroid structures. Some of these newly released structures have even been noted to bud and form elementary-like bodies. *Findings suggest ceroid bodies are derived from vacuolar remnants, related to the vacuole housing the germ.*

By electron microscopy it is difficult to differentiate *Chlamydia* vacuoles from lipid droplets. Both are similar-sized, membrane-bound lucent structures. However, when organisms are present, it is obvious that these structures must be vacuoles. This is an additional explanation to account for the fate of some of the fat in the foam cells: overlooked vacuoles, released from the cell, which go on to form ceroid bodies.

Here again we enter into a controversial area. Some large intracellular lipid droplets in foam cells are overlooked *Chlamydia* vacuoles. Very cunningly camouflaged and hidden among the fat droplets, these go on to form ceroid bodies (Figures 15.15–15.20).

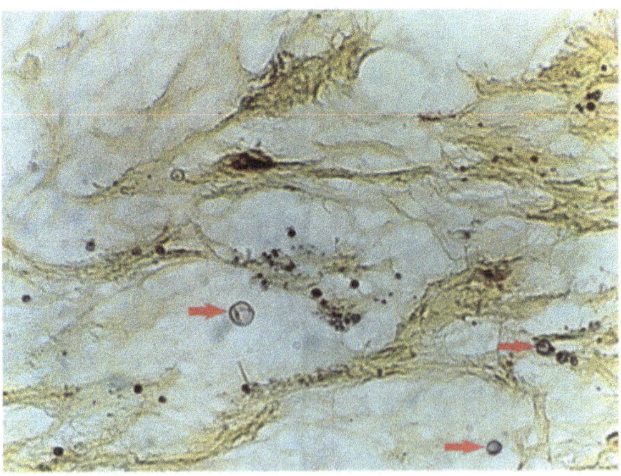

Figure 15.15. Vacuoles in gruel. Micrograph shows clear vacuoles in atheroma gruel (*arrows*).

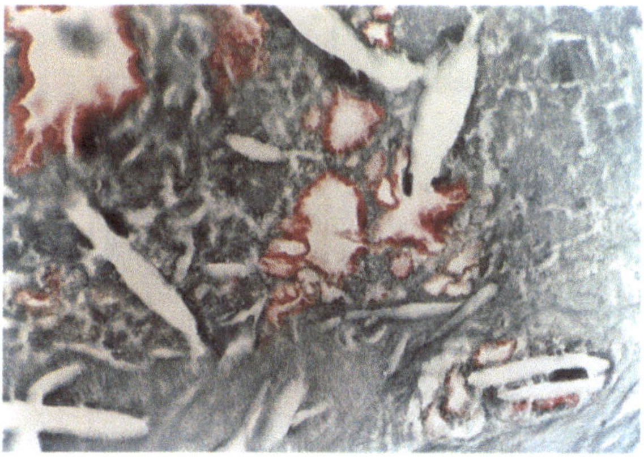

Figure 15.16. Ceroid bodies in gruel. Micrograph shows ceroid bodies consisting of red crenate membranous material in gruel. Masson stain.

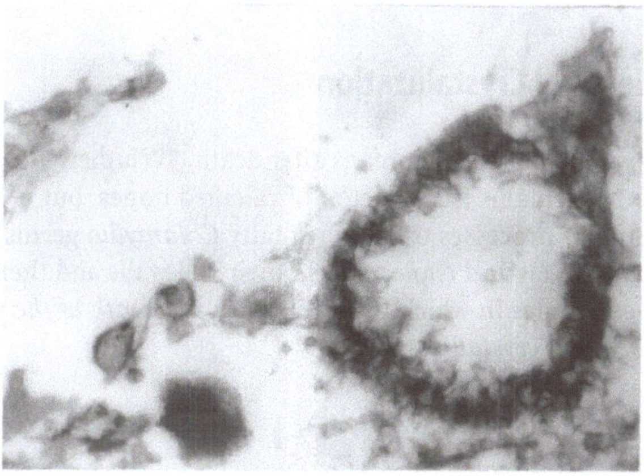

Figure 15.17. Membranous vacuole. Transmission electron micrograph of membranous vacuole and adjacent smaller *Chlamydia*-like elementary structures.

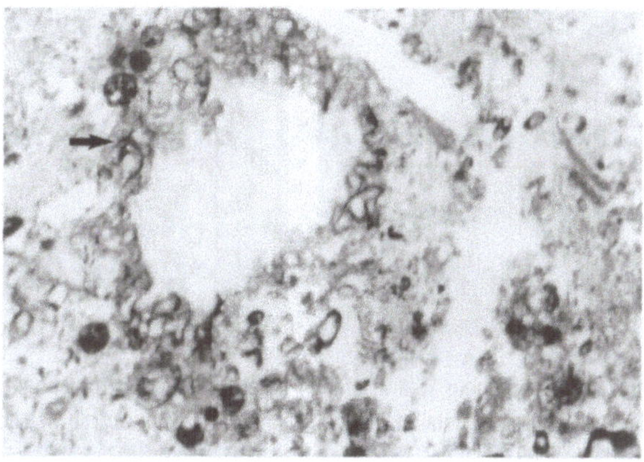

Figure 15.18. Fragmenting vacuole membranous wall. Transmission electron micrograph shows vacuole wall (*arrow*) consisting of multiloculated membranous-type structure breaking up to form small membranous structures.

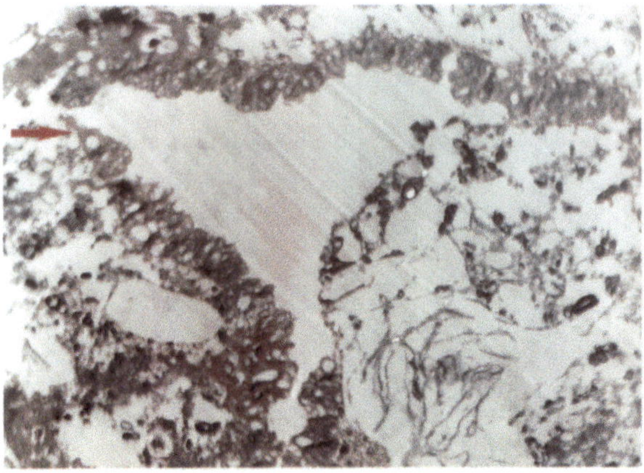

Figure 15.19. Enlargement of vacuole membranous wall. Transmission electron micrograph of vacuole wall seen as wavy loculated multilamellar membranous material (*arrow*).

15.3. Cholesterol Crystallization

We all know what happens to humans after death. "Whither you go? To a place of dust." All that remains is a skeleton of calcified bones, but of the rest there is no trace. Similar processes occur when fatty *Chlamydia* germs and cells die. *Chlamydia* contain fat and cholesterol in their cell walls and there is also cholesterol in the vacuoles in which they live. *With the death of the germs, cholesterol is released and crystallizes out.*

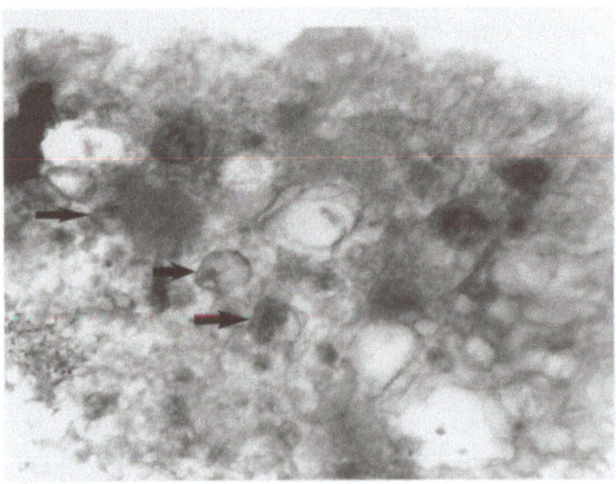

Figure 15.20. Vacuolar membranous wall in greater detail. Electron micrograph shows multilamellar loculated vacuolar wall in greater detail. Elementary forms of *Chlamydia* can be seen interspersed in membranous material (*arrows*).

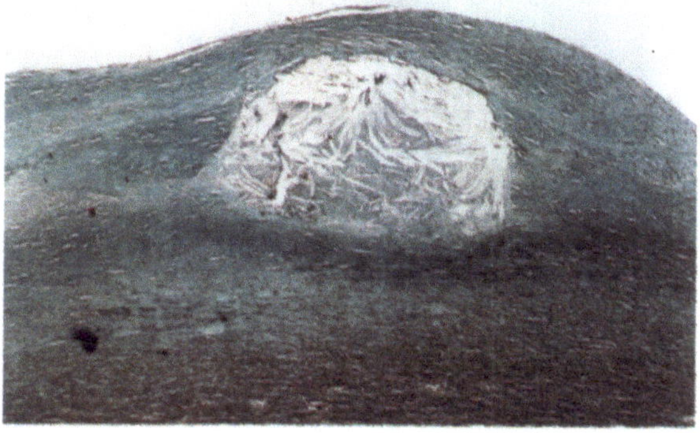

Figure 15.21. Necrotic plaque. Micrograph shows late fibronecrotic plaque consisting of a necrotic core of atheroma gruel and cholesterol clefts. There is overlying fibrotic scar tissue.

There are additional sources of cholesterol in atheroma. *Necrotic muscle cells, macrophages, and red blood cells, which are present in the lesion, all contain cholesterol and other lipids in their cell walls and organelles, which add to the cholesterol crystals.*

Cholesterol crystals are seen as cholesterol clefts with light and electron microscopy and as elongated crystals with scanning electron microscopy (Figures 15.21–15.23).

There has been an idea that if one can determine the origin and formation of the cholesterol, the mysteries of the lesion will be laid bare. Cholesterol represents a group of fats with a vast spectrum of compositional variability, with

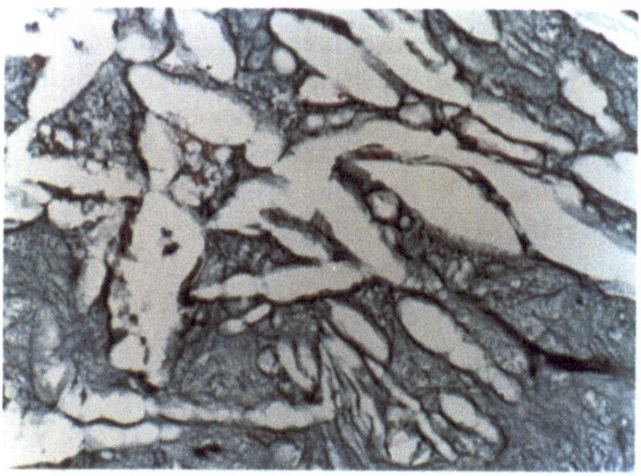

Figure 15.22. Necrotic plaque and cholesterol crystals. Micrograph. Higher magnification of gruel shows clear cholesterol clefts (*elongated clear areas*).

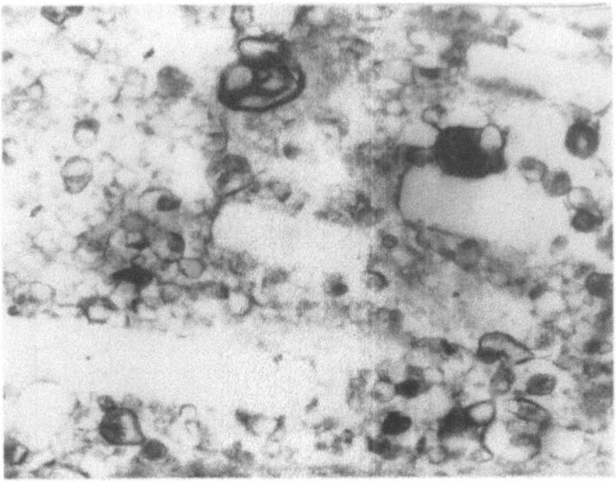

Figure 15.23. Cholesterol crystal in midst of *Chlamydia* germs. Transmission electron micrograph shows atheroma gruel with cholesterol clefts in close proximity to *Chlamydia* (pear-shaped and other structures).

a wide range of physicochemical properties, and with resultant formation of organizational complexity.

There are electron microscopes that have been so highly developed that they are able to magnify to such an extent that it is possible to visualize the structural organization, particularly of the crystalline material and the atoms that go to make up the cholesterol crystals [4].

It is shown that the initiation of cholesterol crystallization comes from aggregation and rearrangement of cholesterol crystals in the amorphous matrix. It was hoped that this information obtained from high-resolution electron microscopic observation of the cholesterol crystals in human atheroma at the atomic level may provide a more complete understanding of the pathogenic mechanisms responsible for the formation of the acellular lipid-rich core. From a biochemical point of view, the cholesterol monohydrate crystals in atheroma are metabolically inert and there is no turnover of crystalline cholesterol in the plaques, suggesting that the crystalline cholesterol is mobilized from an inert metabolic pool of released fat.

Formation and deposition of fat and cholesterol crystals are features of all infectious and necrotic lesions. One has only to look at the cholesterol crystals in the cheese-like fatty material of caseous tuberculosis to appreciate the amount of cholesterol crystals present in chronic infective lesions. The fat and cholesterol in these lesions are derived from inflammatory cells and germs (Figure 15.24).

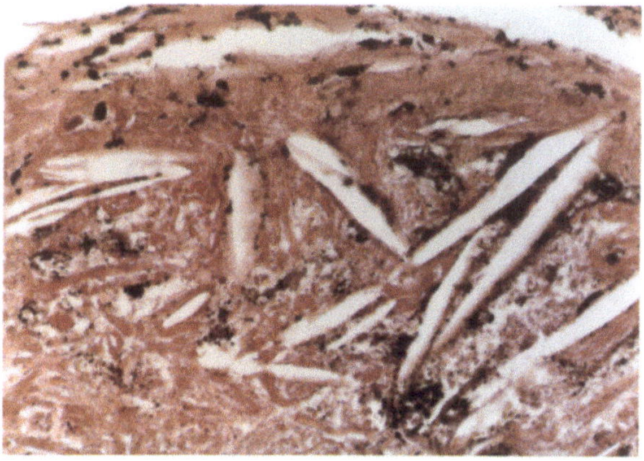

Figure 15.24. Cholesterol crystals in tuberculosis lesion. Micrograph of necrotic tuberculosis lesion with cholesterol clefts (*clear clefts*).

15.4. Late Sequelae: Fibrosis, Calcification, and Angiogenesis

All chronic inflammatory lesions attempt to heal and form fibrous scar tissue. This process also occurs in atheroma, but in this situation, formation of the fibrotic tissue is slightly different. Arteries do not contain the usual scar-forming cells or fibroblasts as in other tissues of the body. Instead, arterial muscle cells become modified and change into myofibroblasts. These cells then have the capability to produce collagen, which goes on to form fibrous scar tissue [5] (Figures 15.25, 15.26).

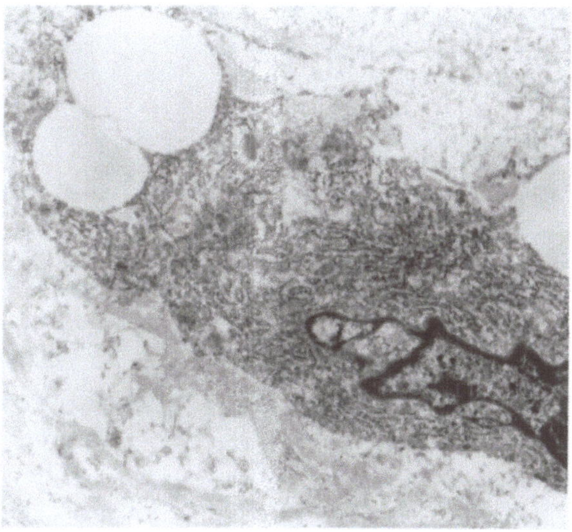

Figure 15.25. Myofibroblast cell. Transmission electron micrograph of myofibroblast cell. The cell contains abundant endoplasmic reticulum in cytoplasm. This is where collagen matrix material is manufactured.

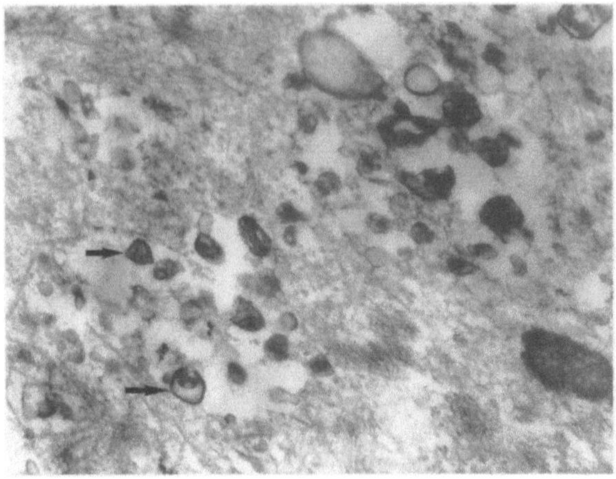

Figure 15.26. *Chlamydia* organisms in scar tissue. Electron micrograph shows collagen or scar tissue, intermingled with *Chlamydia* organisms (*arrows*).

Calcification is another feature of healing. Small foci of calcification occur. Sometimes this can be extensive, involving entire segments of the artery (Figure 15.27).

Part and parcel with any inflammatory lesion comes neovascularization or ingrowth of minute capillaries into the lesion. This mechanism is necessary to convey inflammatory cells to the site of damage. New vessels grow into the damaged tissue; this is called angiogenesis. Sometimes these capillaries can rupture and bleed, resulting in small hemorrhages, effusion of red blood cells,

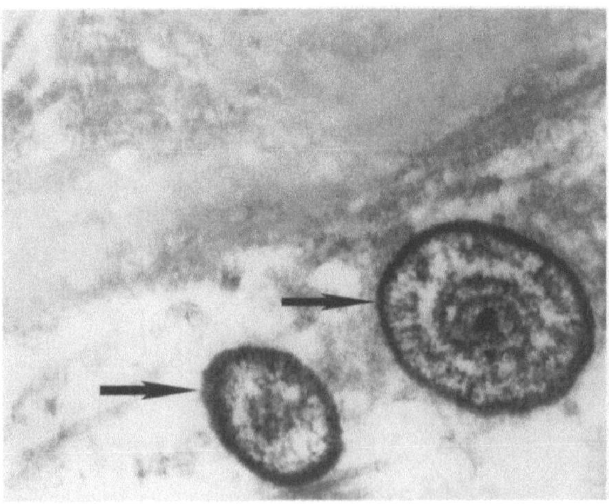

Figure 15.27. Calcification. Transmission electron micrograph shows two foci of calcification in atheroma gruel (*arrows*).

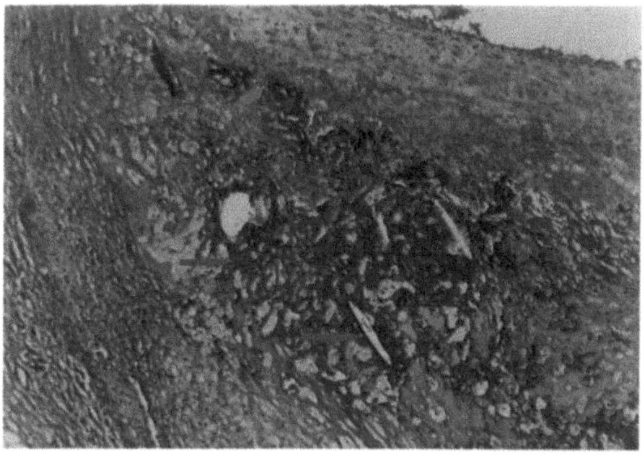

Figure 15.28. Hemorrhage in plaque. Micrograph shows gruel with hemorrhagic area (*arrow*) containing cholesterol clefts (*arrow*).

and iron deposition. If hemorrhage is severe, rupture of the plaque occurs, with extrusion of atheroma into the lumen of the artery, with obstruction of blood flow and dire consequences (Figure 15.28).

References

1. Ball RY, Stowers EC, Burton JH, et al. Evidence that the death of macrophage foam cells contributes to the lipid core of atheroma. Atherosclerosis 1995;114:45–54.
2. Ball RY, Carpenter KLH, Mitchinson MJ. What is the significance of ceroid in human atherosclerosis. Arch Pathol Lab Med 1987;111:1134–1140.
3. Mitchinson MJ, Hothersal DC, Brooks P, et al. The distribution of ceroid in human atherosclerosis. J Pathol 1985;145:177–183.
4. Lee Y-S. High resolution electron microscopic investigation of crystalline cholesterol monohydrate in human atheroma at the atomic level. Micron Microsc Acta 1990; 21(1-2):1–12.
5. Orekhov AN, Andreeva ER, Krushinsky DS, et al. Intimal cells and atherosclerosis. Am J Pathol 1986;125:402–415.

16
Interpretation of Lesion

"A brand-new disease"

16.1. Another Way to Look at the Lesion

Let us look at the lesion in another manner. Scanning electron micrographs do not show the fine detail one sees with transmission electron micrographs, but they do show the scene in three dimensions and are probably more easily related to the world we know.

Scanning electron micrographs show that hordes of small *Chlamydia* organisms attack, overwhelm, and destroy their victims, the poor unsuspecting muscle cells (Figures 16.1, 16.2).

Macrophage scavenger cells clear up the mess. These cells are seen with their tentacles, called pseudopodia, stretching out to grab and engulf the damaged tissue (Figure 16.3).

When the battle is over, all that remains are germs and vacuolar remnants in which the germ once lived (Figure 16.4).

The germs come in a variety of forms and shapes. Some undergo division, multiplication, and budding (Figures 16.5–16.7).

Vacuole remnants are seen as net-like structures (Figures 16.8, 16.9).

As the lesion progresses, cholesterol from cell and germ remnants start crystallizing out to form large crystalline structures. Finally, a mass graveyard consisting of *Chlamydia* germs, cholesterol, cell debris, and red blood cells is all that remains. This is atheroma (Figure 16.10).

With healing comes formation of thick rope-like collagen bundles (Figure 16.11).

The scanning ultrastructural world of atheroma can best be explained by comparing the lesion to happenings in the macro-world, the wild, where game roam freely and where animals attack, kill, and feed off the vegetation and each other. This is nature's way and how animals in the wild get the food they require for survival. One comes across kills and carcasses, and also destruction of grass and trees, not to mention the vast destruction caused by locusts and other

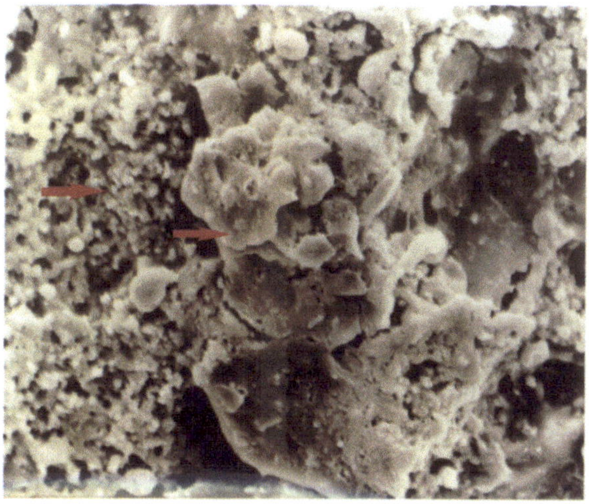

Figure 16.1. Germs attacking muscle cell. Scanning electron micrograph shows multiple small *Chlamydia* organisms (*arrow, left*) attacking and destroying a muscle cell (*arrow, right*).

creatures. In atheroma, it is destruction of muscle cells by germs. Also in nature there are scavengers that play their part by clearing some of the carcasses. There are vultures and then there are smaller creatures, such as worms and ants, which are also nature's way of cleaning up. In the micro-world of atheroma, there are cells that do this work: macrophage cells helped by lymphocytes.

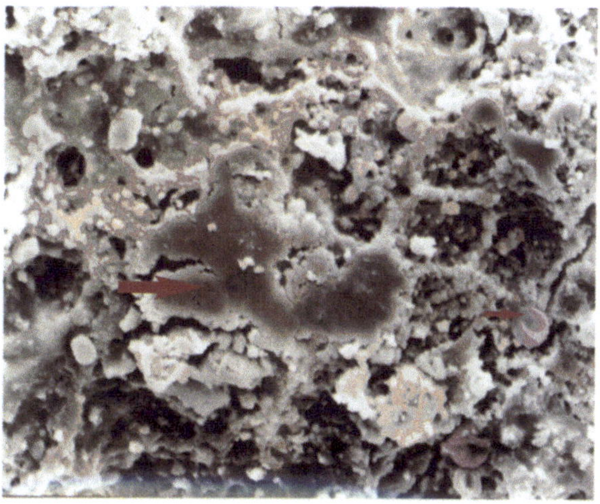

Figure 16.2. Germs and muscle cell remnants. Scanning electron micrograph showing muscle cell remnants (*arrow, left*) with red blood cells (*arrow, right*) and multiple small germ remnants.

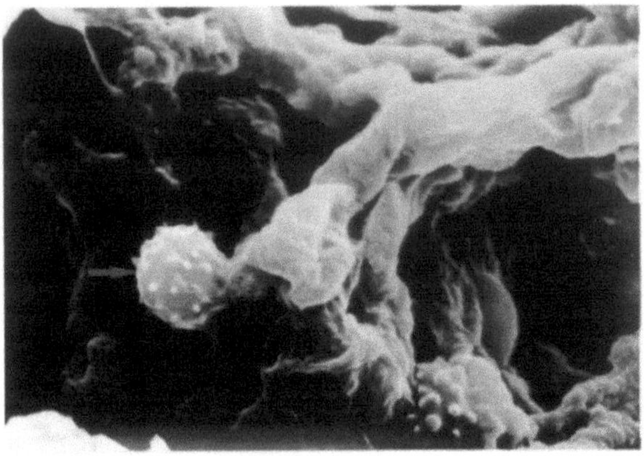

Figure 16.3. Scavenger macrophage. Scanning electron microscopy of macrophage cell with pseudopodia or tentacles to engulf foreign invaders (*arrow*).

Cameramen go in search of wild animals, their habitat, and the way they behave, and take photographs that capture the events. This work is not all that different from the study of lesions and taking of micrographs and electron micrographs. For close-up photographs, telephoto lenses are used to take pictures of animals as they kill and feed off their pray. Marvelous photographs and also irrevocable proof of what happens. Electron microscopes have cameras attached, and one can even attach video cameras to scan the scene. In fact,

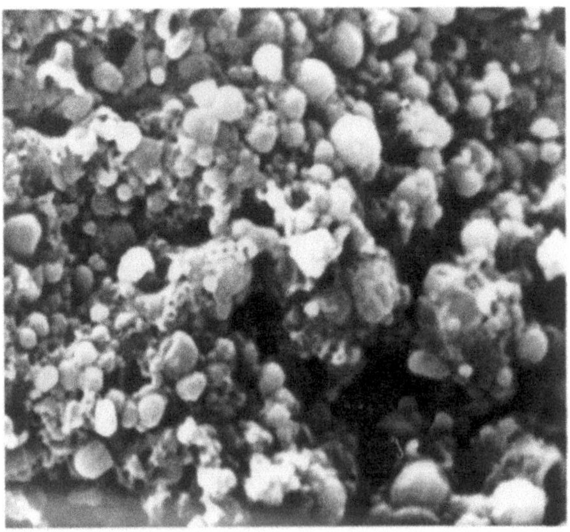

Figure 16.4. Germ remnants. Scanning electron micrograph shows a collection of cell and germ remnants.

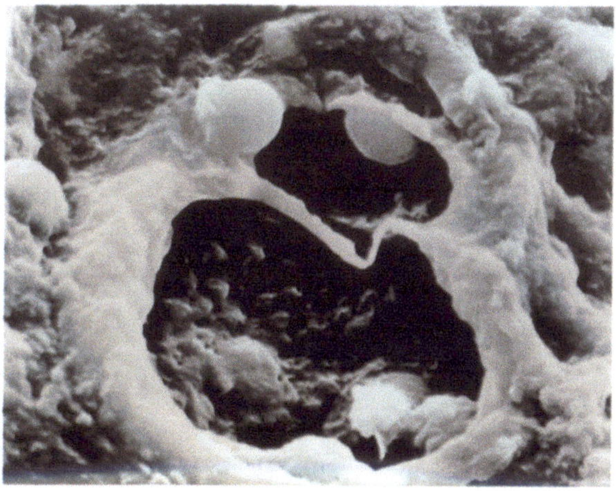

FIGURE 16.5. Germs in vacuole. Scanning electron micrographs of round bodies in vacuole.

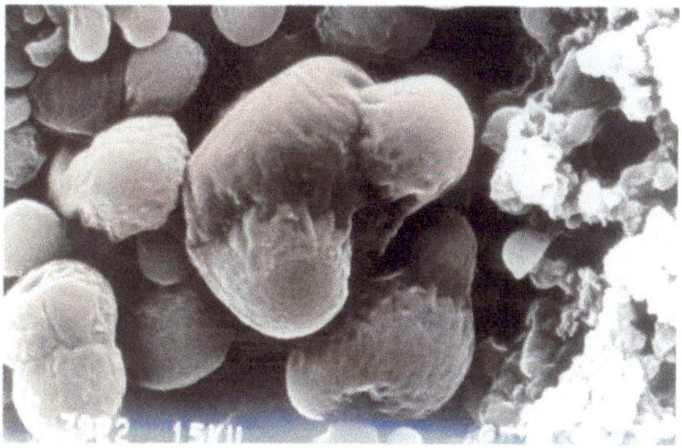

FIGURE 16.6. Dividing germs shown by scanning electron micrograph.

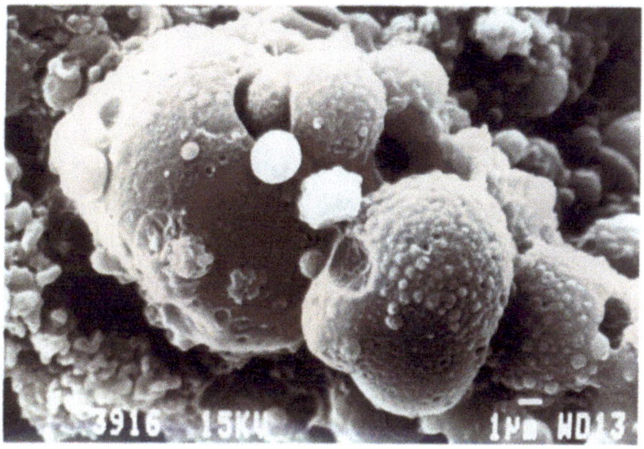

FIGURE 16.7. Budding germs. Scanning electron micrograph shows various forms of growing organisms and budding blebs.

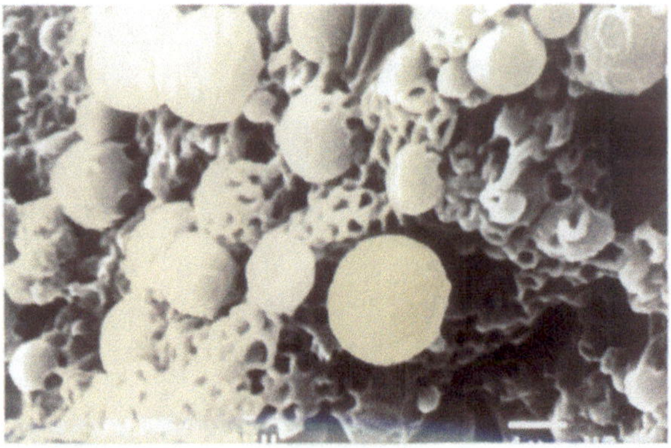

Figure 16.8. Germs and vacuole remnants. Scanning electron micrograph shows round bodies with net-like vacuole remnants.

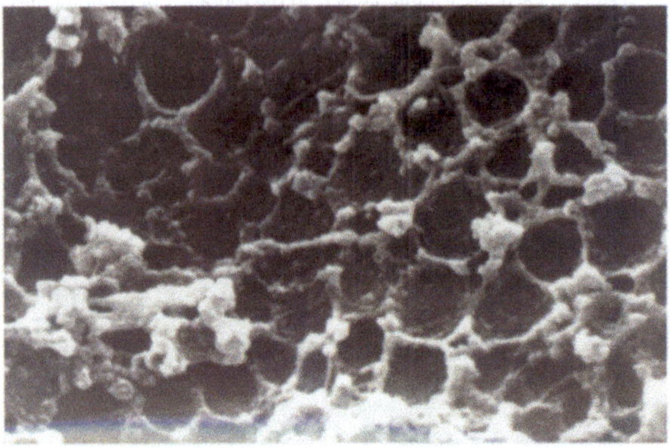

Figure 16.9. Vacuole remnants. Scanning electron micrograph shows net-like vacuole remnants.

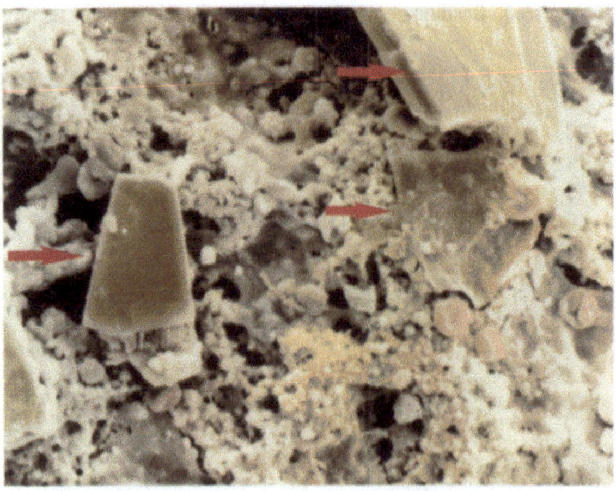

Figure 16.10. Gruel: the end. Cholesterol and germs. Scanning electron micrograph shows the graveyard of cholesterol crystals (*arrows*), germs, and red blood cell remnants.

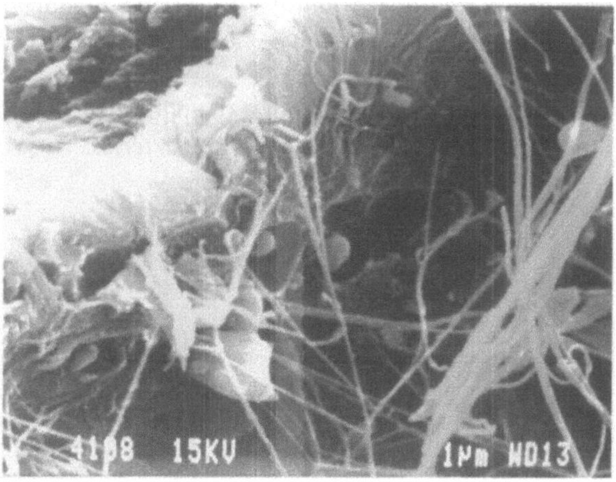

Figure 16.11. Healing scar tissue. Scanning electron micrograph of rope-like collagen bundles.

electron micrographs are much the same as any other photographs. The difference is perhaps that the germs and cells are very small, measured in millimeters and fractions of millimeters, rather than large animals as seen in the wild. Of course, very few persons have seen these ultrastructural details and minute creatures, which are not easily recognized by those who are not electron microscopists or microbiologists.

16.2. Assessment of Evidence

Solving a lesion is much like solving a crime, and as such requires interpretation and assessment of evidence. Coming across a crime in progress, it is fairly obvious what is taking place. However, coming across the scene at a later date, after the event, one has to rely on obtaining leftover evidence, which has to be analyzed and pieced together to ascertain what actually took place.

In the atheroma lesion, there are some cases in which the germs have been caught in the act of destroying muscle cells, but in many cases finding crucial evidence is not so easy. However, if one scrutinizes the arterial lesion, there is usually some evidence that can be found suggesting *Chlamydia* are involved in some manner, either directly or indirectly.

The evidence that has to be considered in assessing the pathological features of the arterial lesion of atheroma is documented in Table 16.1. The features of atheroma are compared to other *Chlamydia* lesions in Table 16.2.

Chlamydia pneumoniae *are not seen as harmless organisms. They are seen to infect, damage, and destroy arterial intimal muscle cells and elicit a macrophage reaction. Early necrotic gruel is viewed as a micro-colony of* Chlamydia *germs formed by proliferation and dispersion of intracellular organisms.* The lesion, when *compared to features of other* Chlamydia *lesions*, shows some similarities.

Based on these factors, it is suggested that the pathological features are consistent with those of a Chlamydia *infection of the arteries.*

TABLE 16.1. New pathological features of atheroma

STAGE	Lesion See references, Chapter 12	New findings See references in Chapters 13, 14, 15
Early	Edematous lesion of Daoud and gelatinous lesion of Daria Haust	Ultrastructurally associated with *Chlamydia* smooth muscle infection and damage consisting of vacuolization with destruction of cytoplasm and myofibrils, and fatty change; this is followed by cellular fragmentation, rupture, release, and dispersion of organisms into extracellular matrix, and loss of intimal muscle cells (see Figures 13.1–13.17).
Fatty streak	Fatty streak lesion viewed as endothelial changes with attraction, adherence, and infiltration ofmonocytes, which change to macrophages, and phagocytose fat to form foam cells.	Viewed as cellular response to damage of muscle cells and germs. Macrophages are seen to engulf and contain not only lipid, but also muscle fragments, *Chlamydia* organisms, and glycogen. Cells coalesce to form multinucleate phagocytic giant cells (see Figures. 14.1–14.8).
Mature plaque	Fibrolipid plaque. Central necrotic core area consists of lipid-rich pool of small membranous lipid droplets, vesicles, dense bodies, and unknown bodies.	Necrotic atheroma lesion consists of central necrotic microcolony of *Chlamydia* elementary bodies and cellular debris. Gruel formed by proliferation of germs with necrosis of foam cells and dispersion of organisms (see Figures 15.1–15.14).
	Ceroid bodies derived from infiltrated lipid.	Ceroid derived from intracellular vacuoles some of which show budding of *Chlamydia* elementary bodies (see Figures 15.15–15.20).
	Cholesterol clefts caused by cholesterol infiltration.	Cholesterol clefts derived from membranes of degenerate germs and cells (see Figures 15.21–15.24).
Late	Fibrosis. Proliferating smooth muscle cells and collagen formation. Apoptosis of muscle cells. Hemorrhage. Fissuring, rupture, ulceration secondary to clot formation	Fibrosis formed as part of attempted healing of chronic inflammatory lesion. Myofibroblastic reaction of attempted healing. Apoptosis of the cells occur after formation of collagen bundles. [Fig 15.25–26] Angiogenesis, as part of healing with neovasularization and granulation tissue formation. Hemorrhage caused by rupture of vessels (see Figure 15.28).

Table 16.2. Comparison of atheroma and *Chlamydia* lesions

	Chlamydia arterial lesions	Other *Chlamydia* lesions
Target cell	Intimal smooth muscle cell	*Chlamydia trachomatis* infections of cervix mucosa, fallopian tube lining cells, trachoma eye epithelium. Lymphogranuloma venereum: inguinal lymph nodes.
Pathogenic mechanism		
Infection of cell cytoplasm	Present	Present
Life cycle in vacuole	Present	Present
Proliferates in vacuole	Present	Present
Necrosis of cell	Present	Present
Release of elementary bodies	Present	Present
Reinfect surrounding cells	Present	Present
Elicits cellular reaction	Present	Present
1. Macrophage	Present	Present
2. Lymphocytes	Present	Present
Necrosis	Present	Present
Fibrosis	Present	Present
Low-grade chronic over years	Present	Present
Complications cause symptoms	Present	Present
Diagnostic inclusion bodies	Present	Present

16.3. What Do We Call the Lesion?

Every disease or lesion should have a descriptive name that identifies it as an entity. The term atheroma, translated literally, means porridge-like hardness, and this is a very nondescript term.

Atheroma is a chronic long-drawn-out infective *Chlamydia* lesion consisting of an infiltrate of monocytes/macrophages and T-lymphocytes. The lesion is also necrotic and fibrotic in nature.

A chronic inflammatory lesion consisting of a compact mass of infiltrating monocyte/macrophage cells with necrosis and fibrosis is a granuloma in pathological terms [1,2].

A more detailed description of the arterial lesion would be "*a chronic infective* Chlamydia pneumoniae-*related arterial granuloma*" or simply "*Chlamydioma*," denoting a compact mass of *Chlamydia* granulomatous material.

References

1. Pickering G. Arteriosclerosis and atherosclerosis. Am J Med 1963;34:7–18.
2. Zumla A, James DG. Granulomatous infection. Etiology and classification. Clin Infect Dis 1996;23;146–158.

17
Confirmatory Molecular Biological Studies

Other evidence

There are molecular biological studies confirming that *Chlamydia pneumoniae* plays some role in the lesion. Studies are unraveling various mechanisms in which *Chlamydia pneumoniae* plays a role in the inflammatory processes, lymphocytic infiltrate, muscle damage, macrophage infiltrate, and other aspects that make up part and parcel of the atheroma lesion [1–32].

17.1. Is Lymphocytic Infiltrate Caused by *Chlamydia*?

In addition to the macrophage infiltrate in atheroma lesions, there is another type of white blood cell, namely, a lymphocyte, that also infiltrates into the artery and helps with the body's defense against the germ.

Examination of atheroma lymphocytes show no pathological changes or *Chlamydia* infection, but there is reason to believe that their presence may be tied to the *Chlamydia* infection in the arteries [5–11].

Various subsets of activated lymphocytes infiltrate into the artery. A type of lymphocyte called the T-lymphocyte is present throughout the life of the lesion and produces a variety of cytokines locally. There is a variety of memory T-lymphocytes, and among these are cells capable of recognizing *Chlamydia* antigens. In an infected plaque, such T-cells may be activated by local antigen and could contribute to the inflammatory process in the arterial wall through CD 40 ligand expression and cytokine secretion [8].

It has also been shown that CD 8 lymphocytes cells are primed by multiple *Chlamydia pneumoniae* antigens, and it is noted increased CD 8 cells are associated with *Chlamydia pneumoniae* in symptomatic carotid plaques [9].

Chlamydia pneumoniae has also been identified as a specific microbial antigen recognized by 41% of the T-cell lines propagated from in vivo activated plaques. *Chlamydia pneumoniae* 60-kDa heat shock protein is also a target for the T-cell immune response.

The molecular biological findings suggest that the lymphocytic cellular infiltrate could well be a response to the *Chlamydia pneumoniae* organisms, and this response may involve autoimmunity [10].

Unstable atherosclerotic plaques contain T-cells that respond to *Chlamydia pneumoniae*. In a subpopulation of symptomatic patients, *Chlamydia pneumoniae* can activate T-cells within atherosclerotic plaques, suggesting that a *Chlamydia pneumoniae*-enhanced proinflammatory response contributes to plaque destabilization in these patients [11].

17.2. Intimal Smooth Muscle Cell Damage

Studies confirm that *Chlamydia pneumoniae readily infect smooth muscle cells* [12]. In addition, vascular smooth muscle cells are shown to express significantly higher levels of gamma-interferon-inducible indolamine 2-3-dioxygenase (IOD) activity than endothelium or mononuclear cells. Because IOD activity is linked to persistent *Chlamydia pneumoniae* infection, this suggests that smooth muscle cells may be an important reservoir of that organism in atherosclerosis [13].

An electron microscopic study has shown that infection with *Chlamydia pneumoniae* induces a spot-like infection in *aortic smooth muscle cells with extensive membrane and organelle damage*. There is chromatin condensation, but no nuclear fragmentation, and chimeric cell death with both apoptotic and necrotic characteristics [14]. Another study has indicated that *Chlamydia induces lipoprotein-induced cell death with necrosis rather than apoptosis* [15]. *Chlamydia pneumoniae* also has other effects on vascular smooth muscle cells, such as activating nuclear kappa B and activator protein 1 [16].

17.3. Monocyte and Macrophage Infiltrate

Chlamydia pneumoniae *induces infiltration and differentiation of monocytes to macrophages in the artery wall and induces foam cell formation* [17,18]. Such infected macrophages may mediate inflammatory changes and are shown to play a role in atherosclerosis and gruel formation [19].

Studies show a role for *Chlamydia* heat shock protein (HSP 60) in the stimulation of immune cells and expression of inflammatory molecules. *Chlamydia pneumoniae* infection of monocytes also plays a role in the induction of extensive changes in the gene expression of the host cell [20].

Chlamydia lipopolysaccharide produces lipid in macrophages by a process of induction and accumulation [21].

17.4. Endothelial Changes [22–27]

As far as the endothelium is concerned, *Chlamydia pneumoniae* triggers a cascade of events that could lead to endothelial activation through various transduction pathways.

Polymorphic membrane protein (PMP) of *Chlamydia pneumoniae* is a proinflammatory mediator in human endothelial cells. The germs also induce proinflammatory mediators and induce transcriptional activation of platelet-derived growth factors in human endothelium cells.

17.5. Collagen Formation [28–33]

Production of the fibroblastic reaction and formation of collagen is shown to be *Chlamydia pneumoniae* related.

There is upregulation of extracellular matrix metalloproteinases and gelatinases in human atherosclerosis infected with *Chlamydia pneumoniae*. Infection produces fibroblast growth factor by smooth muscle cells.

Some studies indicate a potential role for *Chlamydia pneumoniae* in the instability and potential rupture of the plaque [32] and also elastic degradation [33].

These are a few examples of the intricate molecular biological aspects of *Chlamydia pneumoniae* and how they play a role in various processes involved in the atheroma lesion.

References

1. Rupp J, Hellwig-Burgel T, Wolbe V, et al. *Chlamydia pneumoniae* infection promotes a proliferative phenotype in the vasculature through Erg-1 activation in vitro and in vivo. Proc Natl Acad Sci U S A 2005;102(9):3447–3452.
2. Kol A, Bourcier T, Lichtman AH, et al. *Chlamydia* and human heat shock protein 60 activate vascular endothelium, smooth muscle cells and macrophages. J Clin Invest 1999;103:571–577.
3. Kol A, Lichtman AH, Finberg RW, et al. Cutting edge: heat shock protein (HSP) 60 activates the innate immune response: CD14 is an essential receptor for HSP60 activation of mononuclear cells. J Immun 2000;164:13–17.
4. Mayr M, Metzler B, Kiechl S, et al. Endothelial cytotoxicity mediated by serum antibodies to heat shock protein of *Escherichia coli* and *Chlamydia pneumoniae*. Immune reactions to heat shock protein as a possible link between infection and atherosclerosis. Circulation 1999;99:1560–1599.
5. Jonasson I, Holm I, Skalli O, et al. Regional accumulation of T-cells, macrophages, and smooth muscle cells in the human atherosclerosis plaque. Atherosclerosis 1986;6:131–138.
6. Melian A, Geng Y-J, Sukhova GK, et al. CD 1 expression in human atherosclerosis. A potential mechanism for T cell activation by foam cells. Am J Pathol 1999; 155(3):775–786.

7. Ausiello CM, Palazzo R, Spensieri F, et al. 60-kDa heat shock protein of *Chlamydia pneumoniae* is a target of T-cell immune response. J Biol Regul Homeost Agents 2005;19(3–4):136–140.
8. Curry AJ, Portig I, Goodall JC, et al. T lymphocyte line isolated from atheromatous plaque contain cells capable of responding to *Chlamydia* antigens. Clin Exp Immunol 2000;121:261–269.
9. Nadareishvili ZG, Koziol DE, Szekely B, et al. Increased CD8 T cells associated with *Chlamydia pneumoniae* in symptomatic carotid plaques. Stroke 2001;32(9): 1966–1972.
10. Mosorin M, Surcel H-M, Laurila A, et al. Detection of *Chlamydia pneumoniae*-reactive T lymphocytes in human atherosclerotic plaques of carotid artery. Arterioscler Thromb Vasc Biol 2000;20:1061–1067.
11. de Boer O J, van der Wal AC, Houtcamp MA, et al. Unstable atherosclerotic plaques contain T-cells that respond to *Chlamydia pneumoniae*. Cardiovasc Res 2000;48: 402–408.
12. Knoebel E, Vijayagopal P, Figuerora JE, et al. In vitro infection of smooth muscle cells by *Chlamydia pneumoniae*. Infect Immun 1997;65(2):503–506.
13. Sakash JB, Byrne GI, Lichtman A, et al. Cytokines induce indolamine 2–3 dioxygenase expression in human atheroma-associated cell: implications for persistent *Chamydophila pneumoniae* infection. Infect Immun 2002;70:3959–3961.
14. Dumrese C, Maurus CF, Gygi D, et al. *Chlamydia pneumoniae* induces aponecrosis in human aortic smooth muscle cells. BMC Microbiol 2005;5(1):2.
15. Nazzal D, Cantero AV, Therville N, et al. *Chlamydia pneumoniae* alters mildly oxidised low density lipoprotein-induced cell death in human endothelial cells leading to necrosis rather than apoptosis. J Infect Dis 2006;193(1):136–145.
16. Miller SA, Selzman CH, Shames BD, et al. *Chlamydia pneumoniae* activates nuclear factor kappa B and activator protein 1 in human vascular smooth muscle cells and cell proliferation. J Surg Res 2000;90(1):76–81.
17. Yamaguchi H, Haranaga S, Widen R, et al. *Chlamydia pneumoniae* induces differentiation of monocytes into macrophages. Infect Immun 2002;70;2392–2398.
18. Kalayoglu MV, Bryne GI. Induction of macrophage foam cell formation by *Chlamydia pneumoniae*. J Infect Dis 1998;177:725–729.
19. Kuroda S, Kobayashi T, Ishii N, et al. Role of *Chlamydia pneumoniae*-infected macrophages in atherosclerosis development of the carotid artery. Neuropathology 2003;23(1):1–8.
20. Virok D, Loboda A, Kari L, et al. Infection of U937 monocyte cells with *Chlamydia pneumoniae* induces extensive changes in host cell gene expression. J Infect Dis 2003;188(9):1310–1321.
21. Kalayoglu MV, Bryne GI. A *Chlamydia pneumoniae* component that induces macrophage foam cell formation is *Chlamydia* lipopolysaccharide. Infect Immun 1998;66(11):5067–5072.
22. Coombs BK, Chiu B, Fong IW, et al. *Chlamydia pneumoniae* infection of endothelial cells induces transcription of platelet-derived growth factor. Potential link to intimal thickening in a rabbit model of atherosclerosis. J Infect Dis 2002;85(11): 1621–1630.
23. Coombes BK, Mahony JB. *Chlamydia pneumoniae* infection of human endothelial cells induces proliferation of smooth muscle cells via an endothelial cell derived soluble factor. Infect Immun 1999;67(6):2909–2915.

24. Krull M, Klucken AC, Wupperman FN, et al. Signal transduction pathways activated in endothelial cells following infection with *Chlamydia pneumoniae*. J Immunol 1999;162(8):4834–4841.
25. Vilma SA, Krings G, Lopes-Virella MF. *Chlamydia pneumoniae* induces ICAM-1 expression in human aortic and endothelial cells via protein kinase C-dependent activation. Circ Res 2003;92(10):1130–1137.
26. Molestina RE, Millar RD, Ramirez JA, et al. Infection of human endothelial cells with *Chlamydia pneumoniae* stimulates trans-endothelial migration of neutrophils and monocytes. Infect Immun 1999;67(3):1323–1330.
27. Niesser A, Kaun C, Zorn G, et al. Polymorphic membrane protein (PMP) 20 and 8PMP 21 of *Chlamydia pneumoniae* induce proinflammatory mediator in human endothelial cells in vitro by activation of the nuclear factor-kappa B pathway. J Infect Dis 2003;188(1):108–113.
28. Rodel J, Prochnau D, Prager K, et al. Increased production of matrix metalloproteinases 1 and 3 in smooth muscle cells upon infection with *Chlamydia pneumoniae*. FEMS Immunol Med Microbiol 2003;38(2):159–164.
29. Choi EY, Kim D, Hong BK, et al. Upregulation of extracellular metalloproteinase inducer (EMMPRIM) and gelatinase in human atherosclerosis infected with *Chlamydia pneumoniae*. The potential role of *Chlamydia pneumoniae* in the progression of atherosclerosis. Exp Mol Med 2002;34(6):391–400.
30. Kim MP, Gaydos CA, Wood BJ, et al. *Chlamydia pneumoniae* enhances cytokine-stimulated human monocyte matrix metalloproteinases through prostaglandin E2-dependent mechanism. Infect Immun 2005;73(1):632–634.
31. Rodel J, Woytas M, Groh A, et al. Production of basic fibroblast growth factor and interleukin 6 by human smooth muscle cells following infection with *Chlamydia pneumoniae*. Infect Immun 2000;68(6):3635–3641.
32. Lijnen HR. Extracellular proteolysis in the development and progression of atherosclerosis. Biochem Soc Trans 2002;30(2):163–167.
33. Petersen E, Boman J, Wagberg F, et al. In vitro degradation of aortic elastin by *Chlamydia pneumoniae*. Eur J Endovasc Surg 2001;22(5):443–447.

18
Derivation of Lipid in Lesion

Can atheroma lipid be derived from Chlamydia germs?

Lipid has dominated research in the field of atherogenesis—so much so that it has come to be regarded as the sine qua non of atherosclerosis.

There are many different types of lipids or fats present in nature. These substances, an essential part of cells of humans, animals, and microorganisms, form bilayers that make up cell membranes and organelles in addition to supplying nutrition, energy, and performing various other functions. The simplest lipids, called fatty acids, are divided into different types, depending on the length of the structure, the number of carbon atoms, and whether the bonds are saturated. Oleic and linoleic acids are some examples. Phosphoglycerides are another major class of lipid that makes up cell membranes. Cholesterols are also important components of cellular membranes, being part of a larger group of fats called sterols. Waxes are a type of insoluble fat.

It is contended that a diet high in saturated fat or cholesterol correlates with elevated serum cholesterol and an elevated low-density lipoprotein (LDL) level. Raised lipid in the serum is proposed to infiltrate into and deposit in the arterial wall and thus result in the development of atherosclerosis. It is on this basis that atherosclerosis is considered a disease primarily concerned with lipid metabolism and infiltration. However, not everyone agrees with atheroma being a type of cholesterol disease, and in some quarters the hypothesis has been open to some criticism [1]. Actually, the mechanism and the production of lipid in atheroma constitute a very complex process, and *Chlamydia* organisms, may well play a role in this process.

18.1. Atheroma Lipid [1–7]

The normal artery wall contains different lipids, varying in amount from 4.3 mg to 100 mg in children to 10.8 mg to 100 g in the adult [2].

In atheroma lesions, the fat content is greatly increased. In early lesions, *cholesterols, phospholipids, rich in sphingomyelin, and fatty acids such as oleic acid are present. Later lesions contain other fatty acids such as linoleic acid and others including eicosotrienoic acid, which is not found in plasma* [3]. *As the lesion progresses, ceroid, a type of waxy substance* [see Chapter 15: references 2,3], *and hydroxyoctadecadienoic acids, not normally found in mammalian tissue, accumulate* [4,5].

It is postulated that low-density lipoprotein (LDL) particles in the blood infiltrate into the arterial wall. The LDL particles contain a core of cholesteryl esters and triglycerides and a shell containing phospholipids, unesterified cholesterol, and apoB-100 protein. The structures are 22 nm in size, with 1600 molecules of esterified cholesterol, 600 molecules of nonesterified cholesterol, 700 molecules of phospholipids (phosphatidyl choline, 500; sphingomyelin, 200), and 170 molecules of triglyceride, and a single copy of apo-B 100 [6].

It is unclear how exactly these LDL particles infiltrate into the artery wall, but once inside the artery, they are proposed to undergoes a series of remarkable changes involving a variety of different processes. In the artery wall, the particles are proposed to be engulfed by, or infiltrate, both macrophage and smooth muscle cells, where they form large fat globules, measuring from 400 nm up to 1 μm in size, containing 61% esterified cholesterol, mostly of oleic acid.

The cells ultimately disintegrate and release the large fat droplets, which somehow proceed to form a conglomerate of small lipid droplets, 60 to 400 nm in size, which now contain mainly unesterified cholesterol and linoleic acid.. Small lipid droplets also contain 9% phospholipids (compared to 20% phospholipids in plasma LDL particles), as well as sphingomyelin and modified apo-B 100 and apo-E. The particles are further enriched 10- to 50 fold in ceramide (a product of cleaved shingomyelin) compared to LDL particles. There are also products of lipid peroxidation and oxidation, in addition to epitopes against malondialdehyde (MDA)-modified LDL, hydroxynonenal (HNE)-modified LDL, oxidized phospholipid, hypochlorite-modified LDL, and nitrotyrosine.

So, from wherever or whatever the fat is derived, it is not simply the result of straightforward infiltration and deposition of LDL particles from the plasma. If it is indeed derived from the blood plasma, there must be an elaborate mechanism that includes dismantling the LDL globules to enter the artery and building them up to form large intracellular fat globules, high in cholesterol esters and oleic acid. Then, there must be a mechanism that breaks down the large fat globules and then reassembles them to form structures 300 to 400 nm in diameter, high in unesterified cholesterol and linoleic acid [6,7].

However, there are aspects that are difficult to understand. First, some of the fat in the artery, especially the phospholipids, is produced in situ. Second, atheroma contains a variety of fats of composition very different from that of plasma LDL particles. Add the facts that there are some fats not of mammalian origin, some fats not found in plasma, and some ceroid waxy-type fat, and we find ourselves involved in a battery of questions that are not easy to answer.

Another confusing aspect in the equation is the fact that as the lesion progresses the fat changes in content and type.

There are theories and explanation as to how the LDL lipid undergoes these changes in the artery. Included are suggestions that a variety of hydrolytic enzymes and pro-oxidative agents lead to change, breakdown, and reassembly of fat particles. The postulated mechanism is very intricate indeed.

Chymase, tryptase, matrix metalloproteinase, plasmin, kallikrein, thrombin, and lysosomal protease are all postulated to be capable of changing the makeup of the lipid derived from the plasma. Add to this secretory PLA2, secretory SMase, carboxyl ester lipase, cholate, lysosomal acid lipase,15-lipo-oxygenase, myeloperoxidase, heme-oxygenase, nitric acid synthase, NADPH oxidase, ceruloplasmin, transition metals, and other substances, and we have some of the mechanisms that are postulated to be capable of changing the composition of fat in the arteries [6,7].

There also have to be proteolytic, lipolytic mechanisms, phospholipase A2, phospholipasae C, oxidative modification, and cholesterol ester hydrolysis of the particles to form vesicles. Then, there must be molecular mechanisms that cause aggregation of the particles, with suggested interaction and binding of modified LDL to proteoglycans in the presence of lipoprotein lipase [6].

There are questions concerning where exactly all the processes involved are taking place. Also, one could ask why are all these factors present, where do they come from, and what possible reason is there for the artery to change the original fat into a variety of different fats and cholesterols of different content, sizes, and shapes?

Other very pertinent questions are why are the lipid particles membrane bound, why does the lipid contain electron-dense cores, why do the lipid vesicles have the size, shape, and morphology of *Chlamydia* organisms, why can *Chlamydia* be cultured from the fat, and why are the fat content and composition similar to that of *Chlamydia* organisms?

No one has considered the possibility that some of the atheroma lipid could be derived from the *Chlamydia* organisms.

18.2. ***Chlamydia* Lipid** [8–15]

Chlamydia are obligate intracellular organisms that not only use the host's metabolic processes but also require the host's nutrients and lipids for survival. These lipids serve as substrates for supporting growth and also supply essential macromolecular constituents for cellular structure and membranes of the organism.

There are ever-increasing new findings concerning the lipid metabolic processes of *Chlamydia*. The host's phospholipids and cholesterol are trafficked and modified by *Chlamydia* organisms.

It is now shown that host cells infected with *Chlamydia develop a special pathway to transport and incorporate cellular cholesterol and sphingomyelin into the inclusion membrane or the parasitephorous vacuole in which the organism lives.* The process is by a pathway that selectively traffics cholesterol and sphingomyelin from the host cell to the vacuole via the Golgi network. The vacuole represents a unique type of compartment within the trans-Golgi network that incorporates sphingomyelin and cholesterol. Both cholesterol and sphingomyelin are acquired from the host, being derived from LDL particles. In addition, *Chlamydia* are capable of de novo synthesis of phospholipids [8–11]. Of interest is the fact that the sphingomyelin and phospholipids incorporated into the *Chlamydia* vacuoles mimic those of the host cell [12].

Chlamydia also have enzymes to cleave and synthesize triglycerides and various fatty acids [13]. They produce a variety of different straight and branched (iso- and ante-iso-) nonhydroxyl fatty acids, the major one being icosanoic acid. Hydroxy fatty acids are also produced, the most prominent being 3-hydroxyicosanoic acid followed by 3-hydroxy-18-methylicosanoic acid [14,15].

Ceroid is possibly derived from the vacuolar material in which the germ lives. The ceroid appears to be formed in macrophage-derived foam cells and in atherosclerotic lesions, probably derived from extensively oxidized cholestryl linoleate [16,17].

Why do we need to postulate an unexplainable, intricate mechanism for fat alteration and production when cholesterol, sphingomyelin, fatty acid, ceroid, and hydroxyoctadecadienoic acids, a nonmammalian type of fat [4], could all be explainable as being derived from *Chlamydia* lipid?

Some enzymes proposed to be necessary for the production of the various fats in atheroma are also found in *Chlamydia* infections. The secretory phospholipases A2 group 11A (sPLA A211A) are secreted by various cells either continuously or as an acute phase upon stimulation by proinflammatory cytokines. One of their functions is hydrolytic destruction of bacterial membranes. They can also hydrolyze the phospholipid monolayers of high-density lipoprotein (HDL) and low-density lipoprotein (LDL). These also have a tendency to aggregate and produce an enhanced ability to deliver cholesterol to the cells. Lipoprotein lipase gene expression occurs in *Chlamydia*-infected macrophages, and *Chlamydia pneumoniae* associated with sPLA2 expression appears to be an important link between lipid and inflammation [18–20]. An interesting aspect is that glycosamine glycans (GAG) in the presence of lipoprotein lipase are required for lipid vesicle formation in atheroma.

Also, a novel trimolecular mechanism by a heparan sulfate-like glycosamine glycan (GAG) on the surface of *Chlamydia* organisms is required for microbial attachment to host cells. The data suggest that a GAG adhesion ligand mediates attachment by bridging mutual receptors on the host cell surface and on the *Chlamydia* outer surface membrane [21,22]. These facts illustrate that the proposed mechanisms required for vesicle and lipid formation in atheroma are present in *Chlamydia pneumoniae* organisms.

There are thus seen to be many types of lipid in atheroma that are similar to that which occurs in *Chlamydia*, and there are also mechanisms associated with lipid production that can be attributed to *Chlamydia* organisms. In addition, the fat particles are the same size and shape and look like *Chlamydia*.

If viable *Chlamydia* germs are present, then it must also be accepted that these organisms contribute to some of the lipid and also that part of the fat is the result of production, incorporation, and deposition by *Chlamydia* germs.

The formation and deposition of lipid in the lesion is a much more involved process than simple lipid infiltration of serum cholesterol.

18.3. Cholesterol: Friend or Foe?

Cholesterol stands accused of clogging up arteries. As mentioned, in the scientific field there are no trials, no judges or juries, and no conviction of disease-causing criminals. But if there was a trial, the evidence would exonerate cholesterol from any blame and would show that this substance has been unwillingly dragged into and dumped at the site of the clogged arteries. There are many aspects to this debate, and the evidence concerning cholesterol would be so voluminous that it would require a special library building of gigantic proportions to house articles on the subject.

Cholesterol is actually a substance of great value and of vital necessity, playing a role in membrane structure and steroid hormone synthesis as well as in formation of bile acids. As an example of its role in membrane structure, let us look at brain tissue. The brain is a most complex organ, consisting of millions of brain cells or neurones containing much cholesterol in the membranes. Neurones control movements and feelings and allow individuals to think for themselves, among many other functions. If one were to consider where man obtains his thoughts, among various other functions, one would say from his brain. However, this organ has much to be thankful for to the simple cholesterol. Without cholesterol, there would be no brain cells, no brain, and no thoughts.

Not only is cholesterol necessary for brain tissue, but it is also necessary for the formation of hormones so necessary for survival and for continuation of the human species. Think about the function of hormones. Without hormones, no metabolism, no ambition, no moods, no drive, no sex hormones, no continuation of humans. Actually, without cholesterol, humans would be very different creatures from what they are, if they would be there at all.

Now here is the strange situation. Cholesterol does everything for humans and what does it get in return. Contempt, hatred, and being labeled a monster. Something to be attacked and purged from the system.

Cholesterol is an important substance. But rather than viewed in a positive manner, it is seen in a very negative light. Being labeled as a murderous villain does not seem quite fair. The reason for all this negativity is because it is seen as the substance that clogs our arteries, thus causing morbidity and mortality on a gigantic scale.

All this hatred is really unnecessary and quite misplaced. Let us examine the circumstances by which cholesterol is deposited in the artery. From the blood, cholesterol is carried in particles called low-density lipoproteins, known as LDL. Cholesterol as well as other fats use LDL as transporters for their journey. These are fairly small molecules, and how these LDL transporters get from the blood into the arteries is a bit of a mystery. Even though they are small, they have to squeeze through even smaller gaps between endothelial cells that separate the artery from the blood. They keep their route secret, and no one knows how they get there, only to say that they, together with other fatty passengers, do get into the arteries.

Once inside the artery, cholesterol plays a role in various physiological processes and formation of cell membranes. It is also put to use in formation of lipid rafts, floating boat-like structures in the cell membranes. Cholesterol together with other fats called phosphatidyl cholines go toward building these rafts. One of the functions of these rafts is to build platforms for *Chlamydia* to enter the cell [23]. One could perhaps postulate that cholesterol, by virtue of its part in lipid rafts, is necessary and in collusion helps smuggle the nasty *Chlamydia* germs into the muscle cells [24].

Once the cells are infected with *Chlamydia*, the cholesterol, instead of supplying the needs of the cell, becomes waylaid, hijacked, kidnapped, enslaved, and instead of supplying the cell with much-needed fat, supplies the germ with cholesterol. It has been pointed out that *Chlamydia* germs actually block the normal metabolic pathway and waylay the cholesterol at the Golgi complex. There the cholesterol is rerouted and incorporated into vacuoles and elementary body cell walls and also possibly used for nourishment. In this manner, *Chlamydia* use and enslave cholesterol and fats. It is only when *Chlamydia* demise that the cholesterol is able to leave the germ and is set free and crystallizes out. Unfortunately, it is too late. The cholesterol is of no use in this state, and all that remains at this final destination are cholesterol crystals.

If there were a trial, the defending lawyer would present his closing statement something along these lines. Your honor, ladies and gentlemen of the jury, we do not deny my client, the poor cholesterol, is present at the scene of the crime, but we have produced substantial evidence to show that it is an honorable substance of great integrity., essential for human survival. It has been framed, trafficked, and dumped at the site, at the scene of the crime by the true culprits, the nasty *Chlamydia pneumoniae* germs.

References

1. Stehbens WE. The lipid hypothesis and the role of haemodynamics in atherogenesis. Prog Cardiovasc Dis 1990;2:119–136.
2. Woolf N. Lipids and connective tissue of the arterial wall. In: Crawford T (ed) Pathology of atherosclerosis. London: Butterworth, 1982:113–126.
3. Stachowska E, Dolegowska B, Chlubek D, et al. Dietary trans fatty acids and composition of human atheromatous plaques. Eur J Nutr 2004;43(5):313–318.
4. Brooks CJ, Steel G, Gilbert JD, Harland WA. Lipids of human atheroma. Part 4. Characterisation of a new group of polar sterol esters from human atherosclerotic plaques. Atherosclerosis 1971;13:223–237.
5. Garcia-Cruset S, Carpenter KL, Guardiola F, et al. Oxysterols in cap and core of human advanced atherosclerotic lesions. Free Radic Res 1999;30(5):41–50.
6. Oorni K, Pentikainen MO, Ala-Korpela M, et al. Aggregation, fusion, and vesicle formation of low density lipoprotein particles: molecular mechanism and effects on matrix inter actions. J Lipid Res 2000;41:1703–1714.

7. Guyton JR, Klemp KF. Development of atherosclerotic core region. Chemical and ultrastructural analysis of microdissected atherosclerotic lesions from human aorta. Arterioscler Thromb 1994;14:1305–1314.
8. Reynaldo A, Carabeo RA, Mead DJ, et al. Golgi-dependant transport of cholesterol to the *Chlamydia trachomatis* inclusion. Proc Natl Acad Sci USA 2003;100(11): 6771–6776.
9. Wolf K, Hackstadt T. Shingomyelin trafficking in *Chlamydia pneumoniae* infected cells. Cell Microbiol 2001;3(3):145–152.
10. Hackstadt T, Scidmore MA, Rockey DD. Lipid metabolism of *Chlamydia trachomatis*-infected cells :trafficking of Golgi derived sphingolipids to the chlamydial inclusion. Proc Natl Acad Sci U S A 1995;92(11):4877–4881.
11. Wylie JL, Hatch GM, McClarty G. Host's phospholipids are trafficked and then modified by *Chlamydia trachomatis.* J Bacteriol 1997;179(23):7233–7242.
12. Hatch GM, McClarty G. Phospholipid composition of purified *Chlamydia trachomatis* mimics that of eukaryotic host cell. Infect Immun 1998;366(8):3727–3735.
13. Jenkin HM, Makino S, Townsend D, et al. Lipid composition of the hemagglutinating active fraction obtained from chick embryos infected with *Chlamydia psittaci.* Infect Immun 1970;2:316–319.
14. Nurminen M, Rietschel ET, Braude H. Chemical composition of *Chlamydia trachomatis* lipopolysaccharide. Infect Immun 1985;48(2):573–575.
15. Hussein A, Patoprsty V, Toman R. *Chlamydia psittaci* lipopolysaccharide. a reinvestigation of its chemical composition and structure. Acta Virol 1999;43(6): 381–386.
16. Yamada S, Kumazawa S, Ishii T, et al. Immunochemical detection of a lipofuscin-like fluorophore from malondialdehyde and lysine. Lipid Res 2001;42(8): 1187–1196.
17. Hoppe G, Ravandi A, Herrera D, et al. Oxidation products of cholesterol linoleate are resistant to hydrolysis in macrophages, form complexes with proteins and are present in human atherosclerotic lesions. Lipid Res 1997;38(7):1347–1360.
18. Jarros W, Ecky R, Menschikowski M. Biological effects of secretory phospholipase A2 group 11a of lipoproteins in atherogenesis. Eur J Invest 2002;32(6):383–393.
19. Azenabor AA, Job G, Yang S. Induction of lipoprotein lipase gene expression in *Chlamydia pneumoniae*-infected macrophages is dependent on Ca^{2+} signal events. Biol Chem 2004;385(1):67–74.
20. Miya N, Oguchi S, Watanabe I, et al. Relation of secretory phopholipase A(2) and high sensitivity to C-reactive protein to *Chlamydia pneumoniae* infections in acute coronary syndromes. Circ J 2004;68(7):628–633.
21. Zhang JP, Stephens RS. Mechanism of *C. trachomatis* attachment to eukaryotic host cells. Cell 1992;69:861–869.
22. Wupperman N, Hegeman JH, Jantos CA. Heparan-sulphate-like glycosaminoglycan is a cellular receptor for *Chlamydia pneumoniae.* J Infect Dis 2001;184:181–187.
23. Jutras I, Abrami L, Dautry-Varsat A. Entry of the lymphogranuloma venereum strain of *Chlamydia trachomatis* into host cell involves cholesterol-rich membrane domains. Infect Immun 2003;71(1):260–266.
24. Hu H, Pierce GN, Zhong G. The atherogenic effects of *Chlamydia* are dependent on serum cholesterol and are specific to *Chlamydia pneumoniae.* J Clin Invest 1999; 103:747–753.

19
Acceptance

Acceptance of a new pathological entity

19.1. Old Ideas Do Not Change

Based on pathological features, the evidence points to the existence of a *Chlamydia pneumoniae* arterial lesion. The question, however, is whether atherosclerosis lesions are all one and the same, or different lesions, with some being *Chlamydia* related.

Atherosclerosis is a term that is used to describe many different types of lesion. For instance, arterial lesions in experimental animals are all called atherosclerosis. Included in these lesions are Marek's chicken virus, a viral arterial disease with its own special features, also a fatty arterial lesions with large fat-filled foam cells produced by feeding copious amounts of cholesterol to the animal, and fibrotic and healing arterial lesions produced by traumatizing arterial intima. All these lesions are called atherosclerosis, but they are obviously all different lesions. We could ask whether human atherosclerosis lesions are similar. Many different diseases, all culminating in the same fibrotic necrotic end-stage atheroma plaque.

An analogy of such a lesion could possibly be end-stage kidney disease, which is caused by many different types of renal disease. Another lesion would be cirrhosis of the liver, which is the result of different causes, but all of which end in a fibrotic- or cirrhotic-type lesion.

However, the pathological features of the human atherosclerosis lesion suggest that human atherosclerosis lesions are all the same, the reason being that all lesions have consistent, similar features. Edematous lesions, fatty streaks, macrophage lymphocyte infiltrates, same types of fats, similar-appearing vesicles and fat droplets, etc., as outlined in previous chapters. This realization suggests that we are dealing with consistent features and consistent steps that go to make up one type of lesion.

It would also be extremely unusual for different agents to cause the same pathological changes in an artery. Every agent causes its own specific type of damage with its own special pathological features. A stumbling block to acceptance of a *Chlamydia* arterial lesion has been the paucity of histological and electron microscopic studies looking for these types of lesions in arteries. After all, the only way to diagnose and confirm the presence of such a lesion is by actual pathological examination and assessment.

Previous concepts of pathological features of the atheroma lesion have not changed much, even after the finding that viable *Chlamydia* organisms are present in the lesion. Damage to the arterial endothelium is still canvassed as the primary defect. The edematous lesions and damage to muscle cells have not received prominence. Infiltration of monocytes and macrophages is not viewed as a physiological response to muscle damage and germs but rather as an unknown mechanism induced by fat and multiple other injurious substances.

The lesion is still illustrated by a series of drawings conceptualized as small round yellow-colored droplets entering and depositing in the artery to form a lipid core of atheroma. The mature necrotic plaque is accepted as consisting of a lipid pool and not as an area of necrotic gruel-like material with germs. The electron microscopic features of the central lipid core structures have not been studied with a view to comparing them to morphological features of *Chlamydia* organisms grown in culture.

Germs mistaken for lipid is probably a difficult idea to accept. The butter we eat, the fat on meat, the fatty cream in milk, the oily fat that we use for frying, are all fats. One cannot call them anything else. Fat is fat. So who in full possession of their faculties would suggest that the fat in arteries is not fat, but germs. Germs mistaken for fat just does not seem plausible. To suggest that atheroma fat is not really fat is considered ridiculous and nonsensical.

Various other factors also make change difficult. There are some aspects that cannot change suddenly. Research projects are mostly involved in cholesterol and the lipid industry. If atheroma is now accepted as a lesion caused by a germ, do all the research institutes, staff, funding, advertising, etc., simply change direction and start with new types of microbiological research of the lesion?

Changes in direction of research are slow and, in some cases, impossible.

19.2. Rejection of New Ideas [1,2]

Throughout the history of science, and indeed to this very day, new ideas are usually met with skepticism, outright disbelief, and, in many cases, open hostility. In the 1800s Robert Koch, after he discovered the tubercle bacillus, predicted that two generations would pass before his views would be accepted. There were questions as to whether the germ that he had found in the lesion was actually associated with the disease, which was known at the time to be caused by bad humours. He received a lot of opposition and had an uphill battle with his discovery. This is obvious from his comments. He pointed out that in the face of opposition and skepticism it is necessary not to let oneself be tainted by deprecating skepticism and not to let oneself become discouraged.

There have been exceptions. Paul Ehrlich, who discovered chemical chemotherapy agents effective against some microbes, was more fortunate. He did not rock established ideas, but simply discovered an effective chemotherapeutic agent. He said of his discovery, . . . "after years of misfortune, I had one moment of good luck." The original discovery of how the blood circulates through the body, although being profoundly important, was nevertheless a profoundly simple observation and was readily accepted. Harvey, who discovered the circulation of blood, had the supreme fortune to be the right man, in the right place, at the right time.

But this is not the norm. A new discovery goes through a process, a series of rejections, before acceptance finally occurs. Sometimes the process takes years; sometimes the idea is never accepted.

History shows rejections of new ideas are part and parcel of discoveries. Semmelweiss, who suggested that simple washing of the hands with carbolic acid (an antiseptic solution) by midwives and doctors could prevent childbirth-related infection and sepsis, was ridiculed, ostracized, and eventually died in an asylum. Einstein received a few letters a week ridiculing his theory of relativity even until the end of his life. Something about new things means that even if they are correct, seldom are they accepted immediately or even in a lifetime. In actual fact, it appears that the more contrary to current thinking an idea is, the longer and more difficult its acceptance is. It is a fact of life; accepted ideas do not die, even in the face of new evidence.

Arthur Kennedy describes some of the processes of discovery in medicine. There has been, and still is, a fear of challenging authority, or trying to change current views. "It is dangerous to be right in matters on which the established authorities are wrong." There is some difficulty in being open to ideas from a rival camp. He points to the petty jealousies and intolerances of some researchers. Tolerance, and a sneaking suspicion, that others may be right, is not a companion of researchers.

Another aspect of discovery is the slowness of the implementation following new discoveries in medicine. Plank once remarked "a new scientific truth does not win out by convincing its opponents, rather they eventually die off and a whole new generation familiar with the new concept grows up."

References

1. Editorial. Koch's bacillus. Tubercle 1982;63:1–2.
2. Kennedy AC. Discovery in medicine. BMJ 1991;303(6817):1569–1572.

20
Diagnosis of Atheroma Lesions

Looking for new ways to diagnose the lesion

The first aspect that needs attention, if we are to start treatment of atheroma lesions per se, is development of some method of diagnosis.

Diagnosis is a standard requirement necessary in treatment of all lesions. It is imperative to know the exact nature and extent of the enemy, if an attack is to mounted. Without knowledge of these parameters, we are a bit in the dark as to whether treatment is effective. It is not possible to treat the unknown. Not properly, at any rate.

The extent, locality, and size of lesions in the arterial network must be ascertained. Examination of arteries usually does not form part of a general medical checkup, and few if any persons are really aware of the condition of their arteries. Until recently, diagnostic methods have been incapable of showing up the full extent and locality of all atheroma lesions of the arteries. Ultrasound of the carotid arteries, femoral arteries, and aorta offers some information. There are more advanced methods of detection in the pipeline, and it is hoped that in the future accurate assessment of earlier arterial lesions will be possible. With new radiologic studies, clinicians already are being confronted with patients who are showing up with smaller and symptom-less lesions in the arteries.

The next aspect is diagnosing the nature of the lesions. Are they fat-related or *Chlamydia*-related lesions or something altogether different? Every type of lesion requires different treatment. Biopsy is the only way to make a diagnosis, but it is hardly practical to have invasive surgery to obtain a piece of tissue to diagnose symptom-less lesions. Very few persons would agree to such a procedure. This brings out the question as to whether there may be some other more simple methods to diagnose the lesions. Can blood tests be developed to diagnose the lesion of atheroma?

20.1. Serology

Would it not be easy to simply take blood and measure the *Chlamydia* antibody status in the serum and determine if a *Chlamydia* atheroma lesion is present? After all, this is a method of diagnosis that has been used in acquired immunodeficiency syndrome (AIDS) and other viral or infective diseases. Unfortunately, there are some infectious diseases that cannot be diagnosed serologically. First, nearly everyone has been infected with *Chlamydia pneumoniae*, and many people have antibodies in their blood. Also, antibody status does not indicate infection but rather immunity, and there may be cross-reactivity with other *Chlamydia* species.

This situation is much the same as in tuberculosis and other *Chlamydia* infections, where testing of serum does not indicate present infection but only that a person has been in contact with the germ. Also, it has been found that the presence of organisms in the lesion does not bear a relationship to the serological status. In many *Chlamydia* atheroma lesions, persons respond poorly and have little resistance to the germ and have no antibodies in their serum. For these reasons, serology is not used for diagnosis of *Chlamydia* atheroma lesions [1].

20.2. Heat Shock Protein

Human immunoglobulin antibody to *Chlamydia* heat shock protein is associated with coronary artery disease [2]. There are reports that seropositivity appears to be sensitive and unrelated to C-reactive protein and could be a specific marker, but the reports are conflicting in this regard.

20.3. C-Reactive Protein

Raised C-reactive protein (CRP) indicates the presence of nonspecific inflammation, and as such indicates the possibility that *Chlamydia* infection may be present. However, the presence of CRP is not specific for *Chlamydia* and only indicates an infectious state [3,4].

C-reactive protein and complement are hypothesized as major mediators of inflammation in atherosclerotic plaques. It has been ascertained that both complement and C-reactive protein are endogenously generated by arteries. They are 10 fold higher in plaque tissue than in normal arteries. There are intense signals for these substances in smooth muscle cells and macrophages in the plaque, and immunocytochemistry shows colocalization of C-reactive protein and complement. Perhaps a test can be developed to more specifically identify the CRP in atheroma.

20.4. Detection of *Chlamydia* in White Blood Cells and Blood

There are other methods for possible detection of *Chlamydia pneumoniae*. Culturing of blood and looking for *Chlamydia pneumoniae* nucleic acids in blood or in white blood cells are some methods under study [5–7].

20.5. Other Possible Tests

There is also an association between elevated levels of complement, fibrinogen, interleukin 6 (IL-6), and other cytokines [8–10]. These tests may indicate persistent *Chlamydia pneumoniae* infection and a proinflammatory state.

However, none of these tests is specific enough to be used for diagnosis, and at present we are left with pathological examination as the only way to diagnose the lesion.

20.6. Pathological Diagnosis

The problem is obtaining tissue samples, which is restricted to patients who have procedures on their vessels. Other *Chlamydia* lesions such as cervicitis and salpingitis can be diagnosed pathologically, so why not arterial lesions?

The pathological features of *Chlamydia* arterial lesions are outlined in Chapters 13, 14, and 15.

20.7. *Chlamydia* Inclusion Bodies

Chlamydia organisms are very small and can be just visualized with a light microscope at 1000× magnification. The germs have the appearance of fine sand-like granules in the cytoplasm of cells. The presence of *Chlamydia* inclusion bodies, as they are called, is a diagnostic feature of all *Chlamydia* lesions such as lymphogranuloma venereum and *Chlamydia* cervicitis and salpingitis [11–13].

This diagnostic feature has never been described in atheroma previously. Atheroma has been so widely accepted as consisting of fat that persons who have examined the lesion have failed to take note of *Chlamydia* inclusion bodies in the lesion. Text books and articles on the microscopic appearance of atherosclerosis have never mentioned these cells. The late Earl Benditt intimated that he had observed fine granular material in some macrophage cells in atheroma but had been unable to identify the nature of these granules.

Finding the inclusion bodies in cells is a giveaway and a feature that clinches the diagnosis of a *Chlamydia* lesion. *Here is a little more detail on the inclusion material. It is a golden color with hematoxylin and eosin, appears brown with*

Masson's trichrome, pale blue with Giemsa, and gray with the periodic acid-Schiff (PAS) stain, and is positive with specific Chlamydia *immunoperoxidase methods.*

The inclusion bodies are found in smooth muscle cells and macrophages in the vicinity of atheroma gruel.

20.8. Electron Microscopy

Electron microscopy is not usually done routinely, but if it is available this is another method to detect organisms. However, as pointed out, a microscopic search for the germ can only be done on fresh and well-preserved tissue. Search for organisms is extremely time consuming and requires examination of multiple parts of the lesion. The germ is very pleomorphic, occurring in a large variety of different forms and shapes [see references in Chapter 5].

20.9. Immunohistochemical Detection

There are reagents and kits available today to test specifically for *Chlamydia pneumoniae* immunoperoxidase positivity in tissue. Use is made of genus- or species-specific antibodies labeled with peroxidase, or a fluorescent marker is used to identify *Chlamydia* in vascular tissue [14,15].

20.10. Polymerase Chain Reaction

Polymerase chain reaction (PCR) is the method of detection that has been the most widely used but also gives the most variable results [13–16]. The results may vary because of different methodological techniques, sampling of lesion, and amount of organisms present.

20.11. Culture

Culture of *Chlamydia pneumoniae* in atheroma is difficult but has been successfully used in a few specialized centers [14].

References

1. Saikku P. Seroepidemiology of *Chlamydia pneumoniae*-atherosclerosis association. Eur Heart J 2002;23:263–264.
2. Fong IW, Chiu B, Viira E, et al. *Chlamydia* heat shock protein-60-antibody and correlation with *Chlamydia pneumoniae* in atherosclerotic plaques. J Infect Dis 2002; 186(10):1469–1473.

3. Torzewski J, Torzewski M, Bowyer D, et al. C-reactive protein frequently colocalizes with terminal complement complex in the intima of early atherosclerotic lesions of human arteries. Arterioscler Thromb Vasc Biol 1998;18:1386–1392.
4. Yasojima K, Schwab C, McGeer EG, et al. Generation of C-reactive protein and complement components in atherosclerotic plaques. Am J Pathol 2001;158(3): 1039–1051.
5. Blasi F, Boman G, Esposito G, et al. *Chlamydia pneumoniae* DNA detection in peripheral blood mononuclear cells is predictive of vascular infection. J Infect Dis 1999;180:2074–2076.
6. Boman JS, Sonderberg J, Forsberg LS, et al. High prevalence of *Chlamydia pneumoniae* DNA in peripheral blood mononuclear cells in patients with cardiovascular disease and in middle-aged blood donors. J Infect Dis 1998;178:274–277.
7. Sessa R, Di Pietro M, Schiavonni G, et al. *Chlamydia pneumoniae* DNA in patients with symptomatic atherosclerosis. J Vasc Surg 2003;37(5):1027–1031.
8. Bhaki S, Torzewski M, Klouche M, et al. Complement and atherogenesis. Arterioscler Thromb Vasc Biol 1999;19:2348–2354.
9. Toss H, Gnarpe J, Gnarpe H, et al. Increased fibrogen levels are associated with persistent *Chlamydia pneumoniae* infection in unstable coronary artery disease. Eur Heart J 1998;19:570–577.
10. Stenvinkel P, Heimburger O, Jogesstrand T. Elevated interleukin-6 predicts progressive carotid artery atherosclerosis in dialysis patients: associated with *Chlamydia pneumoniae* seropositivity Am J Kidney Dis 2002;39:274–282.
11. Henry MR, de Mesy Jensen KL, Skoglund CD, et al. *Chlamydia trachomatis* in routine cervical smears. Acta Cytol 1993;37(3):343–352.
12. Shiina Y. Cytomorphological and immunocytochemical studies of chlamydial infections in cervical smears. Acta Cytol 1985;29(5):683–691.
13. Swanson J, Eschenbach DA, Alexander ER, et al. Light and electron microscopic study of *Chlamydia trachomatis* infection in the uterine cervix. J Infect Dis 1975;131(6):678–686.
14. Bomen J, Hammerschlag MR. *Chlamydia pneumoniae* and atherosclerosis: critical assessment of diagnostic methods and relevance of treatment studies. Clin Microbiol Rev 2002;15(1):1–0.
15. Dowell SF, Peeling RW, Bowmen J, et al. Standardizing *Chlamydia pneumoniae* assays: recommendations from the Centers of Disease Control and Prevention (USA) and the Laboratory Centre for Disease Control (Canada). Clin Infect Dis 2001;33:492–503.
16. Apfalter P, Blasi F, Boman J, et al. Multicenter comparison trial of DNA extraction methods and PCR assays for detection of *Chlamydia pneumoniae* in endarterectomy specimens. J Clin Microbiol 2001;139(2):519–524.

21
Treatment

Magic bullet or mission impossible

Now we come to the most important aspect of all. Can the new findings lead to formulation of innovative treatments to alter the course of, or possibly even eradicate, the disease?

There are millions of people, in the world at large, who have become victims of this germ and suffer from the disease in one way or another. Heart attacks are a source of a vast number of deaths, not to mention the complications of heart failure and other very uncomfortable symptoms in those who survive. Strokes, with their crippling effects of paralysis of a leg, or an arm, loss of speech, loss of memory, and sometimes loss of general amenities, certainly change a person's quality of life for the worse, and often permanently. Sudden rupture of a large vessel such as the aorta is fatal in many cases. Blockage of the leg arteries with amputation of a limb can be devastating.

The gravity of the situation, and exactly what this little germ is capable of, is illustrated by the following episode, which is not an uncommon scenario. I was once called to the operating theater to examine an atheroma lesion that had been removed from a leg artery during a bypass operation. The patient, a diabetic, had previously had an above-knee amputation of the left leg, because of atheroma, and she was now on the operating table with blockage to the main artery of the other leg. The surgeons were busy doing a bypass operation of the artery in an attempt to restore the blood supply and save the leg. A piece of the blocked artery with atheroma was removed for pathological examination. The artery was badly blocked with atheroma material. I took the atheroma specimen to the laboratory for more detailed examination, where the atheroma lesion was processed and examined by electron microscopy. The lesion contained hundreds of little *Chlamydia* germs. I have often wondered what would have been the outcome if effective antichlamydial treatment were available. Would she have lost her leg and now had the possibility of losing the other leg? Unfortunately, at the time there was, and still is, no standardized, fully effective treatment for *Chlamydia* atheroma lesions. She never received anti-*Chlamydia* treatment, and the question of what her fate would have been had she received effective treatment remains unknown.

21.1. Antibiotic Sensitivity

To start clinical treatment of a new lesion or disease is somewhat of a journey into the unknown. Even though antibiotics may be effective in killing the germs in test tubes, they may not be all that effective in killing the germs in vivo, in living people.

When the antibiotic penicillin was first discovered and tested on human infective lesions, it was found to be ineffective in clearing the sepsis. The dose was initially too small and the treatment too short in duration. Isoniazid (INH), a drug used to treat tuberculosis, did not work all that well when originally tried out on tuberculosis patients. Tuberculosis requires multiple antibiotics and not only INH to be effective.

In the case of atheroma, the best antibiotic to use, possible combinations of antibiotics, and the optimal dose and length of treatment are all unknown entities.

There are various antichlamydial antibiotics on the market. The *Chlamydia pneumoniae* strain isolated from human atherosclerotic lesions has been characterized, and antibiotic sensitivity studies have been done. The germ is sensitive to tetracyclines, macrolides, quinolones, and rifampicin, among other agents. All have a different capability for killing the germ in vitro [1–6].

There are some points to consider in treatment.

Chlamydia pneumoniae *organisms in atheroma usually survive in a persistent, nonculturable, dormant, spore-like form, resistant to conventional antibiotics* [7–11]. In addition, atheroma is a long-drawn-out, chronic granulomatous-type lesion beginning in the early teens and smoldering for many decades. Such lesions are difficult to treat. Examples of these types of lesion are leprosy and tuberculosis, both of which require lengthy treatment, sometimes over years, with a combination of different antibiotics, and atheroma appears to require similar consideration.

For these reasons, there are some problems with treatment of the *Chlamydia* germ in atheroma. It cannot be treated with a short course of antibiotics, as in some other acute *Chlamydia* infections.

Opinions are that treatment of atheroma should be at least 6 months in duration, and possibly with a combination of different antibiotics. Of course, lengthy antibiotic treatment has its own problems, such as side effects and development of resistance to the drugs, but lengthy antibiotic treatment has been used effectively in some chronic diseases such as tuberculosis, leprosy, and acne.

There is also the question that, if we rid ourselves of these organisms, will the lesions and blockage of arteries improve? Will it really be possible for coronary artery disease, strokes, aortic aneurysms, and gangrene of the legs to be treated and cured? All important questions.

21.2. What Happens to the Lesion?

There are different ways by which one can determine the effect of antibiotics on atheroma buildup of the arteries in humans. The easiest way would be to look at the lesion itself. Are germs eradicated with antibiotics? Does the lesion change in size, does it get smaller, and does it disappear after a course of treatment? Does it change in character and heal?

The arteries are hidden from view, and there is no way to observe them continuously during treatment. The only way to visualize the blockage and follow the progress of the lesion is with the use of X-rays and ultrasound examinations [12].

21.3. Does the Lesion Change in Size?

The first attempt to see what happens with antibiotic treatment was simply to undergo an ultrasound of my own arteries, then take a course of antibiotics and follow the size of lesions before and after treatment. I went along to the radiology department and had an ultrasound examination of my neck arteries. As mentioned, everyone has some form of atheroma, and I was no exception. There were indeed some symptom-less atheroma deposits in the neck arteries, as expected. I then took a 6-month course of an anti-*Chlamydia* antibiotic, tetracycline. This course is not as drastic as it appears. This particular antibiotic has been used by dermatologists to treat patients with acne for as long as 2 years in duration.

After the 6-month course of antibiotics had been completed, an ultrasound of my neck arteries was repeated. There was no real change noted in the size of the lesions when these were compared to the original pictures taken before treatment. I waited a further 6 months and repeated the ultrasound again. Still no great changes in size of the lesions. The ultrasound is not all that accurate for precise measurement of atheroma, but at least I knew that after 1 year the size of the lesion did not change greatly or disappear.

Of course, there was a question as to whether the antibiotic, even though effective against *Chlamydia*, did actually reach and kill the germs or change the character of the lesion. The other concern was that I was in my fifties, and from what I had seen, most 50-year-olds usually have scarred, fibrosed, and calcified lesions. End-stage lesions such as these are actually incapable of change and cannot disappear or shrink, so I was really not the person with lesions that were ideal for trying to determine the effect of antibiotics.

I repeated the ultrasound of the neck arteries after 5 years. The lesions were still present, and no great change in size had occurred.

21.4. Does the Lesion Change in Character?

There was a small clinical trial ongoing that examined the effect of anti-*Chlamydia* agents in patients with blockages to the leg arteries. One of the patients in the trial had severe and widespread atheroma and had previously undergone bypass operations for a blocked leg artery and a blocked neck artery. He was now receiving treatment for blockage of another leg artery and also the other neck artery.

In the trial, he had received a 3-month course of antichlamydial treatment, with the antibiotic azithromycin, but in spite of this his neurological symptoms, which were caused by obstruction of the neck artery, did not improve, and he went on to bypass surgery for his blocked carotid neck artery. A portion of the blocked artery was removed at the time of operation and sent for pathological examination.

On examining the artery, it was found that there was very severe obstruction indeed, with complete blockage of a segment of the artery and destruction of most of the artery wall, and the lumen contained an organizing blood clot. It was obvious that damage to the artery was so severe that no amount of healing could possibly change the obstructed and destroyed artery.

The specimen of the artery and blockage was examined in great detail to look to see if any sign of healing had occurred in the atheroma area. The artery was necrotic and scarred, but in the necrotic gruel area *Chlamydia* germs were still present, and a microscopic focus of early granulation or healing reaction was present. So, it appeared that microscopic healing of atheroma was possible. The question was whether this was the result of the antibiotic treatment (Figure 21.1).

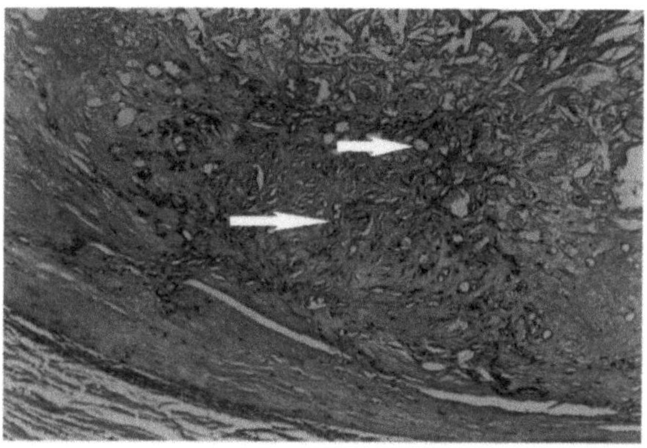

Figure 21.1. Granulation tissue. A microscopic area of granulation tissue or early healing tissue at base of artery (*bottom arrow*). The granulation tissue is in relation to cells with brown sand-like inclusion bodies (*upper arrow*).

References

1. Kuo C-C, Grayston JT. In vitro drug susceptibility of *Chlamydia* strain TWAR. Antimicrobial Agents Chemother 1988;32(2):257–258.
2. Strigl S, Roblin PM, Reznik T. In vitro activity of ABT 773, a new ketolide antibiotic, against *Chlamydia pneumoniae.* Antimicrob Agents Chemother 2000;44(4): 1112–1113.
3. Stewart CE, Coleman K, Mortenson J. Effect of extended pre-incubation with *Chlamydia pneumoniae* and extended incubation with antimicrobials on the minimum inhibitory concentration (MIC) of five antimicrobials. Diagn Microbiol Infect Dis 2001;40:207–209.
4. Cuffini C, Alberto Guzman L, Villegas N, et al. Isolation of *Chlamydia pneumoniae* from atheromas of the carotid artery and their antibiotics susceptibility profile. Enferm Infecc Microbiol Clin 2006;24(2):81–85.
5. Gieffers J, Solbach W, Maass M. In vitro susceptibilities of *Chlamydia pneumoniae* strains recovered from atherosclerotic arteries. Antimicrob Agents Chemother 1998;42(10):2762–2764.
6. Kutlin A, Roblin PM, Hammerschlag MR. Effect of prolonged treatment with azithromycin, clarithromycin or levofloxacine on *Chlamydia pneumoniae* in a continuous-infection model. Antimicrob Chemother 2002;46(2):409–412.
7. Kutlin A, Kohlhoff S, Roblin P, et al. Emergence of resistance to rifampicin and rifalazil in *Chlamydia pneumoniae* and *Chlamydia trachomatis.* Antimicrob Agents Chemother 2005;49(3):903–907.
8. Yamaguchi H, Friedman H, Yamamoto M, et al. *Chlamydia pneumoniae* resists antibiotics in lymphocytes. Antimicrob Agents Chemother 2003;47(6):1972–1975.
9. Gieffers J, Fullgraf H, Jahn J, et al. *Chlamydia pneumoniae* infection in circulating monocytes is refractory to antibiotic treatment. Circulation 2001;103(3):351–356.
10. Hogan RJ, Mathews SA, Mukhopadhyay S, et al. Chlamydial persistence: beyond the biphasic paradigm. Infect Immun 2004;72(4):1843–1855.
11. Krull M, Maass M, Suttorp N, et al. *Chlamydophila pneumoniae.* mechanism of target cell infection and activation. Thromb Haemost 2005;2:319–326.
12. Wendelhag I, Wiklund O, Winklund J. On quantifying plaque size and intima-media thickness in carotid and femoral arteries. Arterioscler Thromb Vasc Biol 1996; 16(7):843–850.

22
Pathological Study

Atheroma lesions are capable of healing

I went on to do a study on pathological features of atheroma lesions in a group of patients who had received an anti-*Chlamydia* antibiotic for at least 6 months duration. The aim was to determine the effect of antibiotics on eradication of the germ and parameters of healing to the lesion [1].

It had been suggested that a pathological study would not be possible. One cannot operate, take a piece of atheroma, give a patient medicine for 6 months, then operate again and take another piece of artery. Such procedures are very invasive and just not done.

Was there any other way to examine treated atheroma lesions? There are some people who receive antibiotics, including macrolides, quinolones, and tetracyclines, for various infections during their lifetime. Some of the agents are also antichlamydial agents. If per chance such people die and come to autopsy, or had bypass surgery, then treated atheroma lesions could be obtained. However, treatment with these antibiotics would have been of short duration, and most likely ineffective in eradicating the germ in a chronic lesion such as atheroma.

There was quite a lot of thought as to which group of persons could possibly have received a lengthy course of antichlamydial antibiotics. Tuberculosis is highly prevalent in South Africa, and treatment for the disease usually consists of a mixture of three different antibiotics [streptomycin, isoniazid (INH), and rifampicin], administered for at least 6 months. Rifampicin is an effective antichlamydial agent in addition to being an antituberculosis agent. Tuberculosis patients, if they die and come to autopsy, would have documented evidence of having been treated with a 6-month course of the anti-*Chlamydia* agent rifampicin. To study these cases, it would be necessary to obtain atheroma lesions from a group of autopsy patients who died of tuberculosis and received rifampicin antibiotic before death. It would also be necessary to examine atheroma lesions from a matched group of autopsy patients who had never received anti-*Chlamydia* treatment for comparison.

Of course, even though the people were dead, there were still some very stringent rules. Authorization to perform the study and consent to use arterial tissue for research purposes had to be obtained from the ethics committee, and other regulations had to be observed. However, after permission was obtained and all regulations had been met, a search for suitable cases to study began in earnest.

Over a period of 8 months, 39 lesions from 17 tuberculosis patients who had received antichlamydial therapy and matched controls of 36 lesions from 23 patients who had not received antichlamydial therapy were collected.

Here are some of the pathological findings.

22.1. Eradication of Germ

Twenty atheroma lesions from each of the treated and untreated groups were stained with monoclonal antibody to identify *Chlamydia* germs in the lesions. Or, more precisely, to determine if *Chlamydia* antigenic remnants were present.

Microscopic examination of the sections showed positive *Chlamydia* antigen staining in 8 of 20 (40%) of the treated atheroma lesions compared to 9 of 20 (45%) of the untreated lesions. Not much difference. *This result indicates that some remnants of the germ are still present even after 6 months of anti-*Chlamydia *treatment.* This does not mean that the organisms are necessarily alive; they may be dead, with only fragments persisting.

The findings are similar to what has been noted in other *Chlamydia* lesions, where complete eradication is difficult and *Chlamydia* remnants persist even after treatment.

A study by Melisano et al. examined the effect of treating patients with the antichlamydial agent roxithromycin for 26 days duration [2]. After 26 days of antibiotic treatment, atheroma plaques were removed at operation and examined for presence of viable *Chlamydia* organisms. Five of 16 treated patients contained *Chlamydia* germs in atheroma plaque, compared to 12 of 16 in non-treated patients. Antichlamydial treatment reduced the *Chlamydia* load but did not entirely eradicate the germs in atheroma [2].

Other studies have ascertained that *Chlamydia pneumoniae* germs survive in blood monocytes and lymphocytes and are not eradicated with use of anti-chlamydial agents [see Chapter 20: references 8, 9]. Studies of treatment of experimental animals have shown persistence of antigenic remnants.

Rifampicin is a very effective antichlamydial agent, but there is a problem in that the germ develops resistance to treatment. Germs are very cunning little fellows. If there is an antibiotic that attacks and kills them, they simply change their metabolism and become resistant to the antibiotic [see Chapter 20: reference 7]. For this reason, tuberculosis and other chronic infections require treatment with multiple different antibiotics. Atheroma lesions probably require similar considerations for germ eradication. Rifampicin combined with a macrolide antibiotic would probably be more effective in eradicating *Chlamydia pneumoniae* organisms [3].

22.2. Size of Lesion

Each lesion was measured microscopically using a special lens, called a graticule, to see if the lesion decreased in size.

The size of the lesions in both the treated and untreated cases were similar. Width and thickness of the treated lesions showed no major differences. This is actually not unexpected. *Granulomatous lesions do not actually change in size, but rather change in character.*

22.3. Stage of Lesion

Each lesion was staged into muscle damage, fatty streak, necrotic plaque, and complicated lesion.

The stages of lesion were similar in both groups studied. *In fact, the stage of a lesion cannot reverse. A late lesion cannot change and revert back to an earlier stage lesion.*

22.4. Decrease in Inflammation

Lesions were examined in detail for amount of cellular infiltrate, which was measured with a graticule.

Decrease in cellular infiltrate indicates a decrease in inflammatory activity. The lesion becomes burnt out and cannot progress further.

The study showed there were an increased number of inactive lesions in the treated group compared to nontreated lesions. In the treated group, 33 of 39 lesions (85%) were inactive, compared to 24 of 36 (67%) of the untreated group.

22.5. Fibrosis and Scar Formation

Healing comprises a number of processes. After the lesion becomes inactive, small blood vessels grow into the damaged area (angiogenesis), and along come the repairmen, called fibroblasts, to repair damaged tissue. Fibroblasts migrate, proliferate, and accumulate at the site of damage. The cells begin to secrete sticky proteinaceous material called extracellular matrix, which is used to repair the damage and fill up the defects. Then this material matures to form tough rope-like strands of collagen material, which eventually form fibrous scar tissue. Afterward, processes akin to interior decorators come to smooth off the rough edges by a process called maturation and remodeling. And so the lesion is healed.

Treated lesions showed some type of healing occurred in 31 of 39 cases (78%), compared to 18 of 36 (50%) of control lesions (Figures 22.1–22.6).

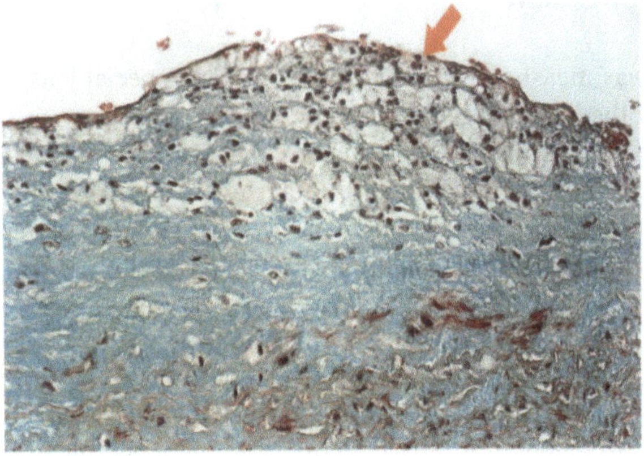

FIGURE 22.1. Fatty streak. Micrograph of fatty streak shows lesion consisting mainly of foam cells (*arrow*).

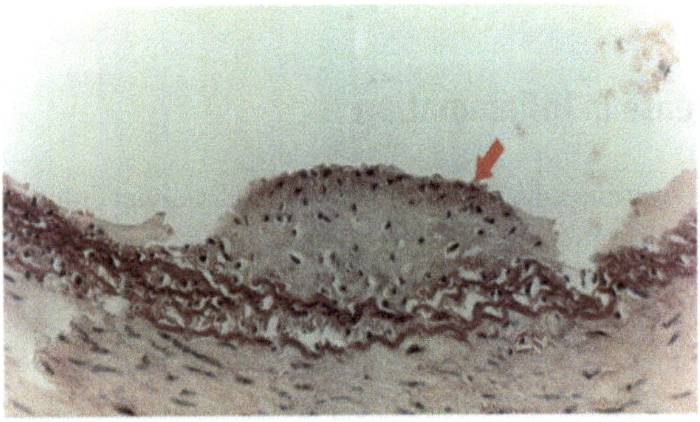

FIGURE 22.2. Healed fatty streak. Micrograph of fatty streak lesion showing healing with fibrous tissue and muscle cells (*arrow*).

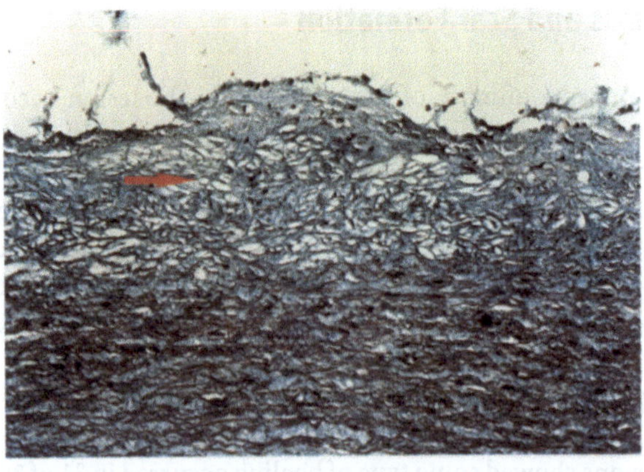

FIGURE 22.3. Necrotic lesion. Micrograph of a necrotic atheroma lesion (*arrow*).

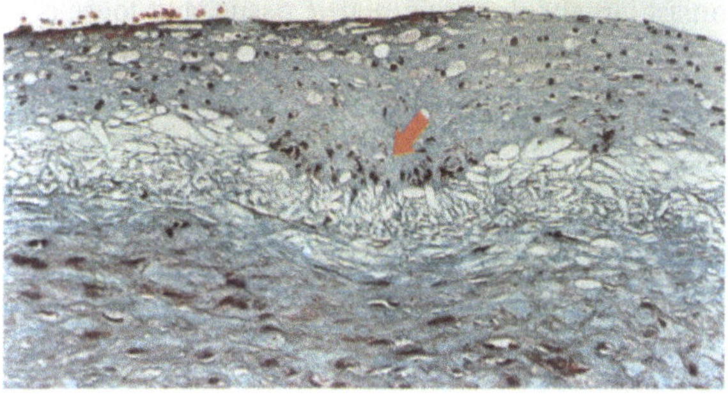

Figure 22.4. Fibroblastic reaction. Micrograph of early healing of atheroma. Fibroblast cells are lined up at site of necrosis ready for action (*arrow*).

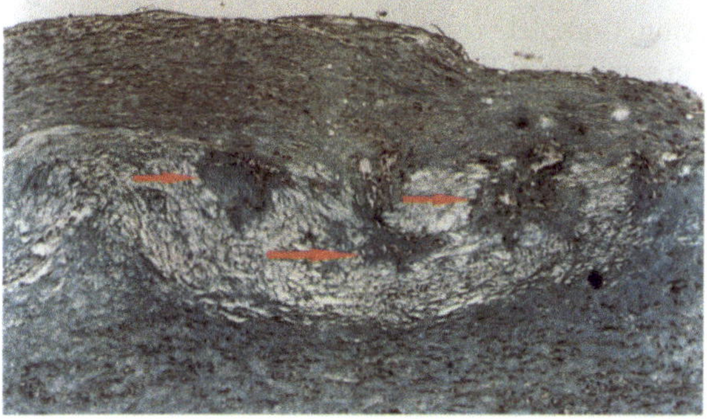

Figure 22.5. Formation of collagen matrix. Micrograph shows fibroblastic cells secreting collagen matrix into necrotic area (*arrows*).

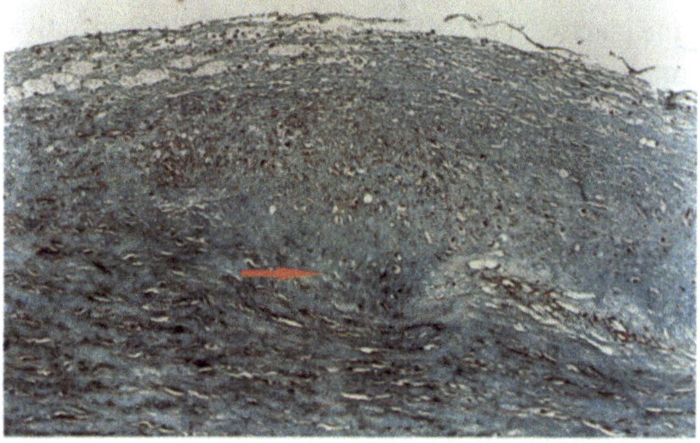

Figure 22.6. Early scar tissue. Micrograph shows maturation of matrix material with formation of collagen and scar tissue, replacing necrotic atheroma gruel (*arrow*).

22.6. Regeneration

Another aspect examined was regeneration of artery components.

Arteries consist largely of muscle, elastic tissue, and loose connective tissue. Interestingly, some of the early lesions that were examined showed the capability to regenerate muscle cell components.

Regeneration of damaged muscle cells is an undescribed feature of atheroma and highlights that healing and regeneration of a very early arterial lesion is still possible, in contrast to more advanced cases, where regeneration of arterial tissue cannot occur.

There was no difference in the number of cases that showed regeneration in the treated as compared to the untreated group.

22.7. Does Treatment Increase Healing?

The question as to what exactly constitutes healing of atheroma has not been clearly defined. Most people believe that healing means shrinkage or disappearance of the lesion. Complete resolution of an inflammatory lesion is, however, only possible in acute cases. If the lesion is chronic, as is the case with atheroma, healing occurs by a process of decrease in inflammation, followed by connective tissue deposition with fibrosis and scar formation [4].

Healing of atheroma is similar to what occurs in other Chlamydia *infective lesions. The lesions do not disappear but heal with fibrosis and scar formation. This is irreversible.*

There is a natural capacity for atheroma lesions to become inactive and heal. In this particular study, 24 of the 36(67%) of the untreated atheroma lesions were inactive and 50% of untreated cases showed some type of healing process.

The major question is whether antibiotics can improve on the healing. The study suggests that treatment with antibiotics may improve the number of healing cases; however, rifampicin or single antibiotic treatment is not fully effective in all cases. Eighty-seven percent of the treated cases, that is, 33 of 39 patients, became inactive, but 6 of the patients still showed active lesions. Also, 31 of 39 lesions showed some healing, but 8 lesions did not heal.

As mentioned, perhaps a combination treatment, as used for other chronic lesions, could prevent resistance and be more effective in eradicating the germ and improve healing.

References

1. Shor A. Studies examining effect of antibiotics on human atherosclerotic lesions. In: Lewis B, Halon DA, Flugelman MY, Gensini GE (eds) Frontiers in coronary artery disease. Bologna: Monduzzi, 2003:55–61.

2. Melisano G, Blasi F, Esposito G, et al. *Chlamydia pneumoniae* eradication from carotid plaques. Results of an open, randomised treatment study. Eur J Vasc Endovasc Surg 1999;18(4):355–359.
3. Wolf K, Malinverni R. Effect of azithromycin plus rifampicin versus that of azithromycin alone on the eradication of *Chlamydia pneumoniae* from lung tissue in experimental pneumonitis. Antimicrob Agents Chemother 1999;43(6):1491–1493.
4. Cotran RS, Kumar V, Robbins SL. Inflammation and repair. In: Robbins pathological basis of disease, 5th ed. Philadelphia: Saunders, 1994:73–89.

23
Other Studies

23.1. Animal Studies [1–6]

Antibiotic studies have been done on experimental animals. There are, however, differences in the pathological features of such lesions compared to humans, and such treatment has been of short duration. Because of this, there has been some criticism of these type of studies. Nevertheless, there were some beneficial effects with the use of the antibiotics azithromycin and clarithromycin. For example, there are studies showing that, in animal models, early treatment with azithromycin prevents development of atherosclerosis lesions, or results in decrease in the size of the lesion. Although antibiotic treatment blunts or eliminates the atherosclerotic response in animals, direct immunofluorescence reveals persistence of *Chlamydia* antigens, and culture-negative DNA is frequently recovered after treatment. These findings question whether complete eradication of the germ occurs with this type of treatment.

23.2. Retrospective Studies [7–10]

One may expect that people who have received antibiotics for various diseases would be less prone to suffer heart attacks. However, the usual course of antibiotics, for a few days only, is probably insufficient to eradicate the germ in the arteries.

Meier et al. [7] did a study to determine whether previous use of antibiotics decreased the risk of developing a first-time heart attack. The study examined a population-based database from the United Kingdom. The case-controlled study examined medical records from a total of 3,315 cases and 13,139 age- and sex-matched controls. A history of patients using antibiotics up to 3 years before the date of an acute cardiac episode was obtained. The results were as follows. Cases that developed cardiac episodes were less likely to have used tetracyclines or quinolone antibiotics, but no such effect with prior use of macrolides, penicillin, or cephalosporin-type antibiotics was noted.

The findings suggest that there is evidence for an association between bacterial infection with organisms susceptible to tetracycline and quinolone antibiotics and risk of myocardial infarction. There was no consideration of duration of treatment, and as it is claimed that macrolides are more effective antichlamydial agents than tetracyclines, the results do not really tally with expectations.

A study at the University of Washington used a database from a large health maintenance organization. The group included 1796 patients and 4883 controls. The findings were that use of erythromycin, tetracycline, and doxycycline during the previous 5 years was not associated with decreased risk of myocardial events. Also, the study found that there was no difference between treatment of 29 days or shorter duration.

In another study, Luchsinger et al. [9] studied a database with 354,258 patients. There were a total of 1,684,091 person-years of observation and 16,139 incidents of myocardial infarction. Findings were that use of anti-*Chlamydia* antibiotics does not reduce the risk of heart attacks.

In a comparative cohort study, 634 users of macrolides and 3827 users of penicillin (a non-anti-*Chlamydia* agent) from the records of the Danish health service registry of prescriptions were followed for 6 months. In the first 3 months, the relative admission for cardiovascular disease was less in patients taking macrolides as compared to penicillin. No effect was noted after 3 months.

All these studies examined patients who had received conventional short courses of antibiotics. This is not really satisfactory treatment to eradicate the atheroma germ or to treat a chronic granulomatous lesion such as atheroma.

23.3. Secondary Prevention Trials [11–35]

There has been widespread interest in treatment of heart attacks and other heart conditions with antibiotics. The Google Internet site contains more than 3.5 million reviews, editorials, studies, lay press articles, etc., on antibiotics and the heart.

Most of the studies on ischemic heart disease are prospective studies that have examined the clinical outcomes of antichlamydial treatment in patients following heart attacks [11–18].

Clinical trials have shown mixed results. For instance, a study on 220 survivors of myocardial infarction who received 500 mg azithromycin (an antichlamydial agent) for up to 1 week showed reduction in future cardiovascular events. This trial has been criticized for the short duration of treatment, which has doubtful effects on eradication of germs in atheroma [19].

Another study examined the effect of a twice-daily dose of 150 mg roxithromycin for 30 days. Patients were followed for 6 months. The rates of severe future events such as recurrent ischemia, myocardial infarction, and ischemic deaths were decreased in this group [20].

The ACADEMIC study did not find a reduction in coronary artery events after antibiotic treatment [21].

A study on the effect of treatment with roxithromycin after coronary stent placement showed a reduced rate of restenosis only in patients with high *Chlamydia pneumoniae* titers but not in patients with normal titers [22].

There are some larger trials on late disease where patients have already suffered heart attacks.

The WIZARD trial screened 7747 participants who were then treated with azithromycin or placebo for 3 months and followed up through the prespecified number of endpoints. Results showed an overall 7% improvement in the treated group of patients; this was not considered statistically significant. There was greater benefit during the initial 3-month treatment period, and as a group diabetics and smokers showed significant reduction in heart attack events. The annualized event rate was 14.6% events for those receiving azithromycin versus 53% in those receiving placebo [28].

The ACES trial of 4000 participants was disappointing in that no difference was found after a year of treatment with the antibiotic azithromycin. Untoward events following a heart attack occurred in 22.3% of those treated with antibiotic azithromycin compared to 22.4% of persons treated with placebo. This was not considered to be statistically significant [29].

The PROVE-IT trial compared one type of statin to another and also examined the effect of adding an antibiotic, gatifloxacin, to the mix. This trial enrolled 4162 patients who had been hospitalized for heart attacks. They were given either atorvastatin or pravastatin, and gatifloxacine was given to half the patients. They were then followed up to see in any of the following events occurred: death, myocardial infarction, unstable angina, revascularization procedure, or stroke [30,31]. Primary events occurred in 26.3% of patients treated with pravastatin, 25.1% of patients treated with placebo, 23.7% of patients treated with the antibiotic gatifloxacin, and 22.4% of patients treated with atorvastatin.

Comparing the results of the two trials (ACES and PROVE-IT), it appears that following a heart attack there is little than can be done. If one goes by the ACES trial results, then taking azithromycin (22.3% complication rate), taking no treatment in placebo group (22.4% complication rate), and treatment with atorvastatin in the PROVE—IT trial (22.4% complication rate) all give similar results. More than one-fifth of patients develop untoward effects. Another aspect is that the WIZARD trial using azithromycin for 3 months appeared to have better effect than the ACES trial using the same antibiotic for 1 year and showed great improvement in diabetic patients and smokers.

These trials look at the effect of treatment in lesions that are probably untreatable to start with. Late calcified, fibrosed, and destroyed arteries are not ideal to see if antibiotics are effective.

23.4. Meta-Analysis [32–35]

Meta-analyses of the trials using antibiotics to treat patients who have had heart attacks showed mixed results. In one analysis, 12 trials with a total of 12,236 patients were included. The overall results were that antibiotics resulted in a nonstatistically significant reduction in the risk of new vascular events or death. In one meta-analysis study, there were 72 patients who did not have coronary heart disease, and these showed a trend for treatment benefit. This finding is consistent with the pathological findings that earlier lesions respond better to treatment than late destroyed arteries, which cannot change.

23.5. Relevance of Clinical Trials

Treatment of heart attacks, depends very much on whether a group of patients show statistical improvement in clinical trials. Trials investigate the percentage of people that benefit from medication in a large groups of subjects. In fact, cardiovascular disease treatment is considered to be one of the most evidence-based disciplines of medicine today. Ronnie Willenheimer has pointed to clinical relevance versus statistical significance in cardiovascular medicine. Methodology, group selection, real-life efficacy, and many other factors versus clinical trial efficacy should be considered in assessing success of treatment [36].

23.6. Unconsidered Aspects

If patients on clinical trials show improvement clinically, this improvement may be the result of pathological change of the lesion, but could also be caused by other factors in the face of unchanged pathology of the underlying atherosclerotic lesion. Conversely, patients may have marked improvement and healing of the underlying atherosclerotic lesion, but this may not be mirrored in the clinical picture.

The antibiotic trials for prevention of secondary events following heart attacks do not assess whether antichlamydial agents kill the germ. Some trials presuppose that antibiotics given in small doses or in an ineffective short course of treatment are capable of eradicating the germ in atheroma.

Studies also accept that eradication of the germ results in improvement of the lesion irrespective of stage. Early-stage lesions appear to be amenable to treatment with possibilities of healing. These lesions are usually in younger persons, and response to treatment in this group should be more favorable. In later lesions, where the damage is more extensive, the situation is different. Only partial healing is possible. Atherosclerotic lesions in patients who have developed symptoms are usually advanced complicated lesions, with organized blood clot in the lumen, and fibrosed and calcified atheroma plaque. These types of lesions are beyond repair and cannot change with treatment.

This situation is similar to other *Chlamydia* lesions, where scarring and fibrosis cannot be reversed. Examples of irreversible *Chlamydia* damage are late-stage trachoma and salpingitis lesions. In these diseases, fibrosis of eye tissue and fallopian tubal tissue is irreparable, even with eradication of the germ. It is too late for treatment.

Not only are some of the late atheroma lesions irreversible, but once a person has suffered a heart attack the heart muscle itself suffers irreparable damage. No amount of healing of the atheroma and restoration of blood supply will regenerate damaged heart muscle. Improved blood supply will not improve the strength of a failing heart. Cardiac arrhythmia, or irregular beating of the heart, will not be changed by healing atheroma. In fact, it is doubtful whether healing of an underlying atherosclerotic lesion of the coronary arteries can greatly alter the clinical course of the disease once established damage to the heart has occurred.

23.7. Noncardiac Treatment Trials

The effect of antibiotics on noncardiac atheroma-related disease also needs investigation, and studies may provide a better indication of the effect of antibiotics on the lesion.

Greater correlation between healing of atheroma and clinical symptoms may come from studies looking at treated noncardiac arterial disease patients. Studies of antibiotic treatment on noncardiac vascular disease exclude many, but not all, of the confounding factors in heart attack patients. For example, in some cases there are secondary organized blood clots in the lumen of atheromatous leg arteries, which would be unaffected by antibiotics.

The greatest bulk of atheroma in the arteries is actually in the aorta, leg, and neck arteries. There have been trials on aortic aneurysms, carotid artery disease, and peripheral vascular blockage [37–41]. Some but not all the trials appear to show a more favorable effect of antibiotics on the clinical outcome. The trials, however, have not been done on a large scale as yet.

References

1. de Kruif MD, van Gorp EC, Keller TT, et al. *Chlamydia pneumoniae* infections in mouse models: relevance for atherosclerosis research. Cardiovasc Res 2005;65(2):317–327.
2. Fong IW. Antibiotic effect in a rabbit model of *Chlamydia pneumoniae*-induced atherosclerosis. J Infect Dis 2000;181(suppl 3):S514–S518.
3. Muhlestein JB, Anderson JL, Hammond EH, et al. Infection with *Chlamydia pneumoniae* accelerates the development of atherosclerosis and treatment with azithromycin prevents it in a rabbit model. Circulation 1998;97:633–636.
4. Muhlestein JB. *Chlamydia pneumoniae* induced atherosclerosis in a rabbit model. J Infect Dis 2000;181(suppl 3):S-505–S-507.
5. Rothstein NM, Quinn TC, Madico G, et al. Effect of azithromycin on murine atherosclerosis exacerbated by *Chlamydia pneumoniae*. J Infect Dis 2001;183:232–238.

6. Shor A. The pathology of *Chlamydia pneumoniae* lesions in humans and animal models. Trends Microbiol 2000;8(12):541.
7. Meier CR, Derby LE, Jick SS. Antibiotics and risk of subsequent first-time acute myocardial infarction. JAMA 1999;281(5):427–431.
8. Jackson LA, Smith NL, Heckbert SR, et al. Lack of association between first myocardial infarction and past use of erythromycin, tetracycline, or doxycycline. Emerg Infect Dis 1999;5(2):281–284.
9. Luchsinger JA, Pablo-Mendes A, Knirch C, et al. Relation of antibiotic use to risk of myocardial infarction in the general population. Am J Cardiol 2002;89:18–21.
10. Ostergard L, Sorenson HT, Linholdt J, et al. Risk of hospitalization for cardiovascular disease after use of macrolides and penicillins: a comparative prospective cohort study. J Infect Dis 2001;1693:1625–1630.
11. Torgano G, Cosentini R, Mandelli C, et al. Treatment of *Helicobacter pylori* and *Chlamydia pneumoniae* infections decreases plasma fibrinogen level in patients with ischaemic heart disease. Circulation 1999;99:1555–1559.
12. Parchure N, Zouridakis EG, Kaski JK, et al. Effect of azithromycin treatment on endothelial function in patients with coronary artery disease and *Chlamydia pneumoniae* infection. Circulation 2002;105:1298–1303.
13. Seamaan HR, Gurbel PA, Anderson JL, et al. The effect of chronic azithromycin therapy on soluble endothelial derived adhesion molecules in patients with coronary artery disease. J Cardiovasc Pharmacol 2000;36(4)533–537.
14. Stone AF, Mendall MA, Kaski JC, et al. Effect of treatment for *Chlamydia pneumoniae* and *Helicobacter pylori* on markers of inflammation and cardiac events, in patients with acute coronary symptoms (STAMINA trial). Circulation 2002;106: 1219–1223.
15. Sinisalo J, Mattila K, Valtonen V, et al. Effect of three months of antimicrobial treatment with clarithromycin in acute non-Q wave coronary syndrome. Circulation 2002;105:1555–1560.
16. Leowattana W, Bhuripanyo K, Singaviranon L, et al. Roxithromycin in acute coronary syndrome associated with infection: *Chlamydia pneumoniae*. A randomized placebo controlled trial. J Med Assoc Thail 2001;84:9(suppl 3):S669–S675.
17. Certec B, Sha PK, Noe M, et al. Effect of short term treatment with azithromycin on recurrent ischaemic events in patients with acute coronary syndrome in the azithromycin acute coronary syndrome (AZACS) trial. Lancet 2003;36:809–813.
18. Zahn R, Schneider S, Friling B, et al. Antibiotic therapy after acute myocardial infarction: a prospective randomized study. Circulation 2003;107:1253–1259.
19. Gupta S, Leathan EW, Carrington D, et al. Elevated *Chlamydia pneumoniae* antibodies, cardiovascular events and azithromycin in male survivors of myocardial infarction. Circulation 1997;96:404–407.
20. Gurfinkel E, Bozovich G, Daroca A, et al. Randomised trial of roxithromycin in non-Q-wave coronary syndromes: Roxis pilot study. Lancet 1997;350:404–407.
21. Anderson JL, Muhlenstein JB, Carlquist J, et al. Randomised secondary prevention trial of azithromycin in patients with coronary artery disease and serological evidence for *Chlamydia pneumoniae* infection (ACADEMIC study). Circulation 1999;99:1540–1547.
22. Neumann FJ, Kastrati A, Miethke T, et al. Treatment of *Chlamydia pneumoniae* with roxythromycin and effect on neointima proliferation after coronary stent replacement (ISAR-3): a randomised, double-blind, placebo-controlled trial. Lancet 2001;357:2085–2089.

23. Grayston JT. Antibiotic treatment of *Chlamydia pneumoniae* for secondary prevention of cardiovascular events. Circulation 1998;97:1669–1670.
24. Grayston JT. Background and current knowledge of *Chlamydia pneumoniae* and atherosclerosis. J Infect Dis 2000;181(suppl 3):S402–S410.
25. Rosen H, Muhlestein JB, Bartlett J, et al. Collaborative multidisciplinary workshop report: clinical antimicrobial trials for primary and secondary prevention of cardiovascular disease. J Infect Dis 2000;181(suppl 3):S582–S582.
26. Shor A. *Chlamydia pneumoniae* atherosclerotic lesions: diagnosis and treatment. In: Lewis BS, Halon DA, Flugelman MY, Hradec J (eds) Advances in coronary artery disease. Proceedings of 4th international congress on coronary artery disease. Bologna: Monduzzi, 2001:33–39.
27. Grayston JT. Antibiotic treatment of atherosclerotic cardiovascular disease. Circulation 2003;107:1228–1230.
28. O'Connor CM, Dunne MW, Pfeffer MA, et al. Azithromycin for the secondary prevention of coronary heart disease. WIZARD Study. JAMA 2003;290:1459–1466.
29. Grayston JT, Kronmal RA, Jackson LA, et al. Azithromycin for the secondary prevention of coronary events. (ACES Trial.) N Engl J Med 2005;352:1637–1645.
30. Cannon CP, Braunwald E, McCabe CH, et al. Comparison of intensive and moderate lipid lowering with statins after acute coronary syndromes. N Engl J Med 2004; 350:1495–1504.
31. Cannon CP, Braunwald E, McCabe CH, et al. Antibiotic treatment of *Chlamydia pneumoniae* after acute coronary syndrome. PROVE-IT Trial. N Engl J Med 2005; 352:1646–1654.
32. Andrews R, Berger JS, Brown DL. Effects of antibiotic therapy on outcomes of patients with coronary artery disease: a meta-analysis of randomized controlled trials. JAMA 2005;293(21):2641–2647.
33. Danish J. Antibiotics in prevention of heart attacks. Lancet 2005;356:365–367.
34. Etiman M, Carleton B, Delaney JA, et al. Macrolide therapy for *Chlamydia pneumoniae* in the secondary prevention of coronary artery disease: a meta-analysis of randomized controlled trials. Pharmacotherapy 2004;24(3):338–343.
35. Illoh KO, Illoh HC, Feseha HB, et al. Antibiotics for vascular diseases: a meta-analysis of randomized controlled trials. Atherosclerosis 2005;179(2):403–412.
36. Willenheimer R. Statistical significance versus clinical relevance in cardiovascular medicine. Prog Cardiovasc Dis 2001;44(3):155–167.
37. Msorin M, Juvonen J, Biancari F, et al. Use of doxycycline to decrease the growth rate of abdominal aneurysms. A randomized double placebo-controlled pilot study. J Vasc Surg 2001;34:606–610.
38. Vanmmen S, Linholt JS, Ostergard L, et al. Randomized double-blind controlled trial of roxythromycin for prevention of aortic aneurysm expansion. Br J Surg 2001; 88:1066–1072.
39. Lindholt JS, Stovring J, Andersen PL, et al. A review of macrolide treatment of atherosclerosis and abdominal aortic aneurysms. Curr Drug Targets Infect Disord 2003; 3(1):55–63.
40. Sander D, Winbeck K, Klingelhofer J, et al. Reduced progression of early carotid atherosclerosis after antibiotic treatment and *Chlamydia pneumoniae* seropositivity. Circulation 2002;106:2428–2433.
41. Wiesli P, Czerswetha W, Meniconi A, et al. Roxythromycin treatment prevents progression of peripheral arterial occlusive disease in *C. pneumoniae*-positive men. Circulation 2002;105:2646–2652.

24
What Do We Know About Treatment of Atheroma Lesions?

Are treatment studies directed against the lesion?

While treatment of heart attack patients has provided some information on the effect of treatment on the clinical outcome, it has not provided sufficient information on the effect of antibiotics on the atherosclerosis lesion per se. There are too many factors involved in causing heart attacks to really specifically pinpoint the exact effect and target of the treatment to the underlying atherosclerotic lesion.

Here follow some factors that specifically target the heart and play a role in heart attacks, and cloud our knowledge of the effect of antibiotics on the atheroma lesion.

24.1. Physiology of the Heart [1]

Every cell in the body needs flowing blood to survive.

The blood carries nutrients and oxygen for the cells and carries away the waste products and carbon dioxide. Both these processes are necessary for cells to survive. The heart is an organ consisting to a large extent of muscle cells and is the organ responsible for maintaining blood flow to the body. The heart, too, needs blood to continue functioning. The muscle cells of the heart cannot survive or function without blood. As all the blood in the body flows through the heart, it would be ideal if the heart could dip into the blood, which is about a third of a cup each beat and five quarts every minute, and absorb whatever it needs. However, the heart wall is fairly thick and is not designed that way. Instead, the heart is nourished by blood from the outside by a system of arteries called coronary arteries, which come off the body's main blood pipe, the aorta. These arteries branch, forming an intricate web of blood vessels, the coronary network.

Here are some interesting facts about this coronary blood supply. The heart consumes 5% of the body blood supply but it makes up only 0.5% of body weight. The heart has a special type of blood supply that is essential for a person to survive. Stop the blood supply to the heart and stop the heart beating, and the body cannot survive. Atheroma, which clogs the arteries, is therefore important in the supply of blood and in supplying the heart with blood, oxygen, and nutrients. What makes the heart prone to suffer a heart attack? The answer lies in the physiology of the heart itself. If anything, the coronary blood supply is very robust. In fact, the heart is able to function well even with partial obstruction to the coronary blood supply. Only when the obstruction becomes so severe that there is no longer any reserve, when the capacity is exhausted, does the heart muscle become needy.

However, if the heart is suddenly called upon to work at maximum effort, it sometimes occurs that the network which supplies the blood cannot deliver the extra blood needed to keep it working at the increased rate. A game of football, sudden effort, a sudden increase in effort. While a young coronary network can easily muster enough reserve to meet the demands of heavy activity, an older one cannot. If the heart is not continually challenged with increased demand, the capacity for reserve becomes more easily exhausted. That is in contrast to other organs in the body. For instance, the blood supply to the limbs works over a much narrower range than the heart and any small deficit gets a response. This does not occur in the heart. If the coronary arteries are to provide a peak amount of blood flow, it is necessary to regularly challenge the supply and create a demand. The key to this demand is physical activity. So, the heart is not simply dependent on the patency of the blood vessels, but other factors also play a role. This understanding should be taken into consideration when assessing the cause of coronary ischemic syndromes and myocardial infarction.

So, although there is underlying atheroma causing obstruction of the blood vessel, additional functional alterations are superimposed on the chronic atherosclerotic lesion in the development of ischemic heart disease syndromes.

24.2. What Causes a Heart Attack? [2,3]

There are factors over and above atherosclerosis that come under consideration in heart attack patients.

Fifty or so years ago the cause of heart attacks were generally accepted as simply atheroma plaque blocking the artery lumen, thus reducing the blood supply to the heart. In the 1960s, with the advent of coronary angiography, it became possible to visualize the coronary arteries during life, and thereafter to monitor the blood flow using invasive and noninvasive procedures. This development allowed a broader view of the pathophysiological mechanisms underlying ischemic heart disease. Clinically different syndromes are recognized: stable angina or pain in the chest with effort; unstable angina with increasing frequency of chest pain; and myocardial infarction, when the decreased blood supply causes damage and death of heart muscle, resulting in scar formation. Atheroma of the arteries is the underlying cause of these syndromes in the majority of the cases. A small number of cases, less than 10%, may have another cause. The degree of blockage is critically important: 75% blockage gives problems in meeting the increased blood supply needed for increased demand, 90% reduces blood supply even at rest. There are other factors, such as length of lesion, multiplicity of lesions, perfusion pressures, and variables that influence myocardial demand. There is a general observation of a strong correlation between the extent and severity of anatomic disease and clinical syndromes of ischemic heart disease. However, there is no question that in many patients symptoms may occur in the presence of severe triple vessel disease, double vessel disease, single vessel disease, or even insignificant atherosclerotic disease, which has emphasized that there are dynamic changes in arteries other than simple occlusion of the lumen.

While the underlying pathology may be the atheroma, there are other factors that play a role in decrease of blood oxygen supply to the heart and its effects. Some of the factors that can decrease the blood supply and oxygen-carrying capacity follow. Oxygen is carried by the red blood cells in the blood. Anemia causes a decrease in the red blood cells. High altitude, lung disease, and smoking all cause a decrease in oxygenation of the blood, as do infections and disease of the lungs.

Then there are nerves that supply the arteries and can cause the arteries to dilate or constrict. Added to this are chemical mediators that affect the arterial tone and arterial patency. In some cases, there may be some degree of spasm of the artery, causing a decrease in lumen and so influencing the blow flow.

There are also diseases that affect the blood flow through the arteries. An occlusive thrombus can block the lumen, or small aggregations of platelets can block the smaller arterial branches supplying the heart muscle. A number of clotting factor abnormalities can cause increased clotting of the blood, and so decrease the blood flow through the arteries.

There are also diseases that increase the blood viscosity, and this has a similar detrimental effect on blood flow. Dehydration makes the blood thicker and less easy to flow. Sludging occurs where the red blood cells stick together and the blood cannot flow so easily through the arteries.

The arterial wall itself can become damaged and roughened, impeding the flow of blood on the arterial surface and so slowing flow of blood through the arteries to the heart muscle.

All these factors can compromise the blood and oxygen supply to the heart.

24.3. Atherosclerosis Is Not the Same as Ischemic Heart Disease

Coronary arteries make up but a small part of the total arterial vasculature, and atheroma of these arteries contribute only a small amount toward the total atheroma bulk in an individual. The total degree and amount of atheroma in the vasculature does not correlate with ischemic heart disease. Also almost everyone from the late teens onward has some form of atheroma in their arteries.

Articles mix and interweave cardiovascular heart disease and atheroma and portray both as one disease. Atheroma may cause symptoms of ischemic heart disease, or strokes, but these symptoms are not an indication of the extent or severity of lesions. *A meta-analysis on ischemic heart disease is not a study of atherosclerosis, and it has been pointed out that there is a 20-fold difference in incidence of factors associated with ischemic heart disease and atherosclerosis.*

Atheroma is a widespread vascular disease and should not be viewed as only playing a role in cardiovascular disease. It should be considered as a pathological entity that affects all arteries and requires its own special diagnosis and treatment.

References

1. Zamir M. Secrets of the heart. Sciences 1996;36:26–31.
2. Buja LM, Willerson JT. "Variant" angina": One aspect of a continuous spectrum of vasospastic myocardial ischemia. Am J Cardiol 1978;42:1019.
3. Willerson JT, Hillis LD, Winniford M, et al. Speculation regarding mechanism responsible for ischemic heart disease syndromes. J Am Coll Cardiol 1986;8(1):245–250.

25
Other Treatment Possibilities

Looking for new treatments

There are an increasing number of articles showing that existing drugs may have beneficial effects on the atheroma lesion.

25.1. Statins [1–7]

Hydroxy-3 methylglutaryl-coenzyme A (HMG-CoA) reductase inhibitors, or statins, constitute the most powerful class of lipid-lowering drugs [1–3]. However, there is reason to suspect that the beneficial effects and decrease of heart attacks may be caused by other factors than lowering of serum lipid, as some studies show benefits of statins independent of the lipid-lowering effect [4].

There are a few possible avenues by which the statins could act. Statins may have beneficial effects because of their antiinflammatory properties, their effects on cellular membranes, and may even possess anti-*Chlamydia* properties.

The most frequently proposed model is that statins interrupt proinflammatory signaling by blocking geranyl-geranylation of proteins such as Rho and Ras in a way that influence their activity. In vitro studies have demonstrated simvastatin, atorvastatin, and cerivastatin downregulate the mRNA expression for cytokines (IL-6, IL-8, monocyte chemotactic protein) in the endothelium and leukocytes. Also, statins significantly reduce C-reactive protein and tumor necrosis factor-alpha. Both pravastatin and cerivastatin reduce macrophage content of atherosclerotic lesions and simvastatin, fluvastatin, and atorvostatin reduce inflammation and suppress tissue factor and metalloproteinases. Statins also reduce adhesion factors of the disease, and also natural cells, T-cell proliferation, and monocyte chemotaxis.

Statins can also change the structure and function of cell membranes. For instance, the response of lymphocytes to exogenous signals such as antigens is orchestrated by a number of molecules that cluster in cholesterol-rich areas of the cell membrane known as cholesterol or lipid rafts. Lipid rafts act as platforms that bring together molecules essential for the activation of immune cells, and also separate such molecules when the conditions for activation are not appropriate. There is some evidence that inhibition of cholesterol synthesis by statins disrupts the lipid rafts and thereby influences the function of lymphocytes. Because of this, statins may have a favorable effect on sepsis and may even have effects on transcription and replication.

An effect that has not been greatly considered is the fact that *Chlamydia* require cholesterol containing lipid rafts in the host cell membrane in order to enter, infect, and become internalized in host cell's. Statins disrupt these lipid rafts and this inhibits entry, uptake and infection of *Chlamydia* organisms in arteries.

Another effect of statin drugs is the reduction of macrophage-*Chlamydia pneumoniae*-mediated signaling and transmission [5]. Statins could therefore reduce cell interaction and activation. Statins also modify the inflammatory response of human macrophages and endothelial cells infected with *Chlamydia pneumoniae* [6].

Even more surprising are studies showing that statin drugs have an effect on the *Chlamydia* germ itself. Simvastatin treatment causes lowering of viable *Chlamydia pneumoniae* counts in mice [7].

25.2. Aspirin [8–10]

Aspirins have a beneficial effect on patients with ischemic heart disease. They are stated to prevent future untoward events after a heart attack and to decrease the incidence of heart attacks in high-risk patients. The mechanism by which they act is suggested to be modification of thrombus formation, that is, decreasing the chance of forming blood clots that block the arteries. Clot busters is a term that has appeared in the literature.

Aspirins have other possible mechanisms that may have a direct role on the lesion. There are NF-κB transcription factors that are in turn involved in a variety of cellular genes that regulate the inflammatory response. NF-κB is sequestrated in the cytoplasm by inhibitory proteins, IkB, which are phosphorylated by a cellular kinase complex known as IKK. IKK is made up of IKK-alpha and IKK-beta. Aspirin and salicylates act by their specific inhibition of IKK-beta, thereby preventing activation of NF-κB related genes involved in the inflammatory response [8].

Also, aspirins, strangely enough, are shown to have an anti-*Chlamydia* effect by actually inhibiting *Chlamydia* growth through NF-κB-mediated gene expression. This is a crucial step in the developmental cycle of *Chlamydia pneumoniae* and may account for the cardioprotective activity of aspirin. This anti-*Chlamydia* effect of aspirin occurs in concentrations as low as 10^{-4} mol/L (a concentration commonly achieved by therapeutic doses of aspirin in humans) [9,10].

25.3. Antihypertensive Agents [11,12]

There are studies showing that use of antihypertensive agents may also have beneficial effects for heart attack patients.

The reason for possible benefit is not known, but of relevance could well be the fact that atheroma lesions occur only in high-pressure areas of blood vessels. The main artery from the heart, the aorta, has the highest pressure and is worst affected by atheroma, then leg arteries, neck arteries, arteries to the heart, etc. The arteries to the lungs are of lower pressure and do not develop atheroma, unless the pressure becomes raised by pulmonary hypertension, as it is called; only then does atheroma occur. Atheroma does not occur in veins, which are low-pressure areas. However, if veins are transplanted into arteries with resultant increase in pressure, then atheroma occurs in the transplanted veins.

The effect may be the result of physical forces, but a point to consider in trying to explain this phenomenon is the fact that *Chlamydia* germs require high pressure to infect cells. For cell cultures to be infected with *Chlamydia* germs, the culture plates have to be centrifuged to increase the pressure. This is necessary to physically infect and drive the *Chlamydia* organisms into the cells. Is this the reason for the beneficial effect of antihypertensive agents in decreasing the incidence of heart attacks? Maybe lowering the blood pressure with antihypertensive agents decreases the capacity for *Chlamydia* to infect arteries.

25.4. New Innovative Agents [13,14]

Nowadays, with all the chemotherapeutic agents and antibiotics that are around, perhaps there is a possibility of looking into other drugs that may be effective in eradicating the *Chlamydia* organism.

There is an observation that may hold a clue to use of agents other than antibiotics. Autopsy cases show that cancer patients who have received chemotherapy appear to have less severe atheroma lesions. With loss of weight, and decreased cholesterol and fat, what do you expect, they say. But perhaps there is another factor. Chemotherapy. Can this treatment rid the body not only of malignant cells but also *Chlamydia* germs? Too radical. Paul Ehrlich, who discovered some agents to eradicate germs more than a hundred years ago, said, of the agents he was testing: Drugs slaughter microbes, and when it does not kill them it tames them. However, there are problems. The drugs do outlandish things to the human body, so much so that one would say they were lies if you heard the queer things they can do.

One cannot treat patients with drugs that have severe side effects.

Discussions with oncologists suggest that it may be true that patients under treatment with chemotherapy appear to suffer fewer heart attacks, strokes, aortic aneurysms, and peripheral vascular disease. Also, bypass and stents appear to be less necessary. Scanty articles in the literature suggest that ischemic heart disease in postmastectomy patients is decreased, and tumor patients have decreased incidence of heart attacks.

There is little literature on the effect of chemotherapeutic agents on *Chlamydia* germs. However, there are some articles indicating that interferons, fluorouracils, possibly the antibiotic chemotherapeutic agents, and other cytostatics used in the treatment of tumors may be effective in eradication of *Chlamydia* germs.

To give some indication of the processes and difficulties involved in looking into this aspect and maybe finding an effective new medication for this disease, one would first have a well-controlled study to ascertain how great the statistical decrease of atheroma in patients receiving chemotherapy really is. It would be then be necessary to find the most effective drug and how it can be modified to produce a safe, easily administered tablet that would be effective in the treatment of the atheroma lesion. A long-drawn-out exercise.

25.5. Immunization [15–17]

This type of treatment has and is being investigated. It should be pointed out that trials will take many years for results. Effective vaccines, however, have not been developed or shown to be beneficial in other *Chlamydia* lesions, and an attempt to find an effective vaccination for people against a form of blindness caused by *Chlamydia trachoma* has been unsuccessful. A vaccine is still not in use, and 30 years of effort have failed to produce an effective *Chlamydia* vaccine for humans. The prototype vaccine, which works in mice, holds out hope that a vaccine to combat infection may still be developed.

The problem is that that people who shake off one bout of *Chlamydia* infection, either naturally or with antibiotics, are just as susceptible to the next episode, because the immune system rapidly forgets how to recognize the *Chlamydia*. This failure is in contrast to other infections in which an infection elicits a lifelong immunity from reinfection by that particular agent. The surface of *Chlamydia* does not contain proteins that are distinctive enough to draw the full fire of the immune system. This is one of the reasons that have wrecked previous attempts to make substrates of vaccines based on coat proteins. To develop a more effective vaccine, focus has been extended to include substances in the cell wall, or other substances recognized by the immune system. The vaccine, if it could be given in pill form, would certainly be a breakthrough. However, as yet there is no effective vaccine, and this type of treatment remains in the realm of research [17].

References

1. Sheperd J, Blaw GJ, Murphy MB, et al. Pravastatin in elderly individuals at risk of cardiovascular disease (PROSPER) randomized trial. Lancet 2002;360:1623–1630.

2. Volpe M, Tocci G. Integrated cardiovascular risk management for the future: lessons learned from the ASCOT trial. Aging Clin Exp Res 2005;17(4 suppl):46–53.
3. Libby P, Aikawa M. Stabilization of atherosclerotic plaques: new mechanisms and clinical targets. Nat Med 2002;8(11):1257–1262.
4. Kurata T, Kurata M, Okada T. Cervastatin induces carotid artery plaque stabilization independently of cholesterol lowering in patients with hypercholesterolaemia. J Int Med Res 2001;29:329–334.
5. Dechend R, Gieffers J, Dietz R, et al. Hydroxymethyl glutaryl coenzyme A reductase inhibition reduces *Chlamydia pneumoniae*-induced cell interaction and activation. Circulation 2003;108(3):261–265.
6. Kothe H, Dalhoff K, Rupp J, et al. Hydroxymethyl glutaryl coenzyme A reductase inhibitors modify the inflammatory response in human macrophages and endothelial cells infected with *Chlamydia pneumoniae*. Circulation 2000;101(15): 1760–1763.
7. Erkkila L, Jauhiainen M, Laitinen K, et al. Effect of Simvastatin, an established lipid-lowering drug, on pulmonary *Chlamydia pneumoniae* infection in mice. Antimicrob Agents Chemother 2005;49(9):3050–3062.
8. Yin MJ, Yamamoto Y, Gaynor RB. The anti-inflammatory agents aspirin and salicylate inhibit the activity of I kappa B kinase-beta. Nature (Lond) 1998;396:77–80.
9. Tiran A, Gruber HJ, Graier WF, et al. Aspirin inhibits *Chlamydia pneumoniae*-induced nuclear factor kappa-B activation, cytokine expression, and bacterial development in human endothelial cells. Arterioscler Thromb Vasc Biol 2002;22(7): 1075–1080.
10. Yoneda H, Miura K, Matshushima H, et al. Aspirin inhibits *Chlamydia pneumoniae*-induced NF-kappa activation, cyclo-oxygenase-2 expression and prostaglandin E2 synthesis and attenuates *Chlamydia* growth. J Med Microbiol 2003;52:409–415.
11. Fox KM. EUROPA Study. Lancet 2003;362:782–788.
12. Schartzkopf B. Repair of coronary arteries after treatment with perindopril in hypertensive heart disease. Hypertension 2000;36:220–251.
13. Pehrsson SK, Linnersjo A, Hammar N. Cancer risk in patients with ischaemic syndromes. J Int Med 2000;258(2):124–132.
14. Hossain MS, Easmin S, Islam MS, et al. (2004) Novel thyocyanato complexes with potent cytotoxic and antimicrobial properties. J Pharm Pharmacol 2003;56(12): 1519–1525.
15. Coghlan A. Shapely vaccine targets: *Chlamydia*. New Sci 1996;152:18.
16. Makela PH. Is cardiovascular disease preventable by vaccination? Ann Med 1999;31(1):61–65.
17. Christianen G, Pedersen A-S, Hjerno K, et al. Potential relevance of *Chlamydia pneumoniae* surface proteins to an effective vaccine. J Infect Dis 2000;18(suppl 3): S328–S337.

26
Conclusion

This book is about the *discovery and pathology of a new infectious arterial lesion.*

Micrographs and electron micrographs show h*ow a germ infects and destroys our arteries.* The focus is on new findings and pathological features: arterial muscle cell damage, foam cells phagocytosing not only fat but also muscle fragments and germs. A novel look at atheroma gruel formation by a process of infection and destruction of cells with proliferation and dispersion of germs is shown. Diagnostic criteria are discussed.

There are important practical questions. How do we get infected? *When* does infection occur? *Who* is infected? *What* is the extent of the infection?

And, can we diagnose the lesion clinically?

Most important of all is treatment. To treat or not to treat: that is the question. *Will* it be possible to find really effective anti-*Chlamydia* treatment and eradicate the disease completely? *Will* the goal of no more heart attacks or strokes become a reality?

Acceptance of the lesion is a first step in starting to look for some form of treatment or solution. The fact that we are living with a deadly infective germ may not be very pleasant, but let us console ourselves that knowing the extent of disease in our arteries and what we are cohabiting with is better than not knowing and living in ignorance.

It is hoped that some type of effective treatment will be found in the future: Treatment that will eradicate these little fellows, purge them from our arteries, kill them totally and completely before they kill us.

Glossary of Terms

Artery: A tube of muscle and elastic fibers lined with endothelium that transports blood from heart to capillaries
Atheroma: Fatty material that blocks arteries
Atherosclerosis: Disease that causes obstruction of vessels
Binary fission: Division of germs into two equal parts
Blood: Consists of plasma fluid and blood cells
Epidemiology: Study of the distribution of disease
Etiology: Science of the cause of disease
Extracellular: Tissue outside cells
Fatty streak: Term used to denote small yellow flecks of early atheroma
Genetics: Study of cellular chemistry involving genes
Hyperlipidemia: Increased fat
Immunological: Reaction of the body in overcoming various injurious agents
Infectious: Invasion by organisms causing disease
Inflammation: Series of changes in reaction to injury from various causes
Lesion: Local disease condition
Macroscopic: Features as seen with naked eye
Matrix: Tissue in which cells are embedded; primitive collagen
Membranes: Fatty structures enclosing outer cell
Metabolism: The process by which chemical substances carried in the blood derived from nutrients are digested, broken down, and renewed
Microorganism: Organisms seen with aid of light microscope
Microscopic: Features as seen with use of a light microscope.
Molecular biology: Molecular processes of the cell and disease
Monoclonal: Antibody against a single antigen
Morphology: Study of structure of organisms
Plaque: A word used to denote mature lesion of atheroma
Plasma: Blood without blood cells
Proteonomics: Study of formation of proteins by genetic material
Serum: Fluid remaining after blood has clotted
Species: A subdivision of genus
Sporulating: Multiplication of multiple organisms in a vacuole or sack
Strain: Subdivision of species
Vacuole: A clear space in a cell
Vascular: To do with blood vessels
Vein: A vessel carrying blood from capillaries back to heart
Vesicles: Small membrane-bound sac

Index

MIX
Papier aus verantwortungsvollen Quellen
Paper from responsible sources
FSC® C105338

If you have any concerns about our products,
you can contact us on
ProductSafety@springernature.com

In case Publisher is established outside the EU,
the EU authorized representative is:
Springer Nature Customer Service Center GmbH
Europaplatz 3, 69115 Heidelberg, Germany

Printed by Libri Plureos GmbH
in Hamburg, Germany